Excellent book. It provides an easy to understand guide for both practitioners as well as patients. It is succinct, to the point and destined to become an instant classic!

—Daniel Kessler, D.O., ABFM, ABIHM
Primary Care & Functional Medicine

Three Steps to Superior Health *offers rarely-seen insight into the importance of balancing mind, body, and emotions to achieve vibrant health. Dr. Gutierrez offers practical methods to achieve this goal, which will help in many aspects of life, not only diet. He teaches you meditation methods for stress management that will keep you mentally honed to take up the challenges of changing your diet.*

—Janice Stanger, Ph.D.
Author of *The Perfect Formula Diet*

It is such a relief to see a health professional both recognize and implement a program which has the power to save millions of lives and turn around our health-care, or, more appropriately, a sick-care system that is costing us billions of dollars. This wonderful book covers the three most important lifestyle factors: stress management, diet, and exercise. Dr. Gutierrez takes you from generalized goals such as "be happy," "get fit," or "lose weight," or "how do I heal myself?" to a concrete, step-by-step plan. And we all know where failure to plan gets us. With this book in hand, you can confidently reach these goals. I'd recommend it to all who want to see improvements in their own health as well as everybody else's!

—Ruth E. Heidrich, Ph.D., Ironman Triathlete
Author of *A Race For Life, CHEF, Senior Fitness,* and
Lifelong Running

This book is so inspiring. The presentation of meditation is wise and practical. The integration of different aspects of health and scientific research is powerful. WOW!

—Rev. Judith Elia, M.S., LMFT
Minister of Unity of Oroville

Dr. Gutierrez strikes gold! This book is a perfect blend of science and practicality guiding the reader step by step to a healthier life. He offers simple but powerful tools that place vitality within our reach and awaken our higher selves. Thank you, Dr. Gutierrez!

—Lin Silvan, Executive Director
Eugene Veg Education Network

Dr. Gutierrez provides an empirically based manual for achieving superior health that is strongly grounded in research yet rendered accessible by his use of both professional and personal illustrations. His unique manual is founded on reducing stress—a prominent contributing factor in many physical and mental conditions—through mindfulness and meditation. As documented in the psychological and neuroscience literature, these practices can help reduce stress, alleviate depression and anxiety, decrease the effects of trauma, and improve one's overall sense of well being. He builds upon this groundwork of stress reduction by integrating the benefits of a plant-based diet while also presenting a sustainable approach to movement and exercise. Dr. Gutierrez is a prominent leader among medical providers, helping people to live healthier, more fulfilling lives in body, mind, and spirit. This book is a must-read for anyone seeking improved health and well-being.

—Ericka Souders, Ph.D., L.P.C., N.C.C.
Counselor, Educator, and Supervisor
Licensed Professional Counselor

THREE STEPS *to* SUPERIOR HEALTH

An Evidence-Based Guide
for Stress Reduction,
Longevity, and Weight Loss

ORESTES GUTIERREZ, D.O.

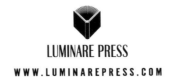

LUMINARE PRESS
WWW.LUMINAREPRESS.COM

Three Steps to Superior Health
An Evidence-Based Guide For Stress Reduction, Longevity, and Weight Loss
© 2015, Orestes Gutierrez, D.O.

Printed in the United States of America

Cover Photo: George Filgate
Cover Design: Claire Last
Back Cover Author Photo: John Freshwater

Luminare Press
467 W 17th Ave
Eugene, OR 97401
www.luminarepress.com

LCCN: 2015956630
ISBN: 978-1-937303-70-9

I dedicate this book to my wife, Pamela, and three children, Sofi, Maria Rose, and Boone for their unyielding patience, support, and love throughout the writing of this book.

A special thanks to my mother, whose unconditional love and support allowed me to chase my dreams and realize that the sky is the limit.

Contents

Part Three

Movement in
Moderation is Your Fountain of Youth

Foreward

I AM THANKFUL I HAD THE PRIVILEGE OF MEETING Dr. Gutierrez in medical school where he was already educating me on the benefits he talks about in his book. Today he continues to be an inspiration. He not only educates, but he truly lives every aspect of what he preaches. His writing brings me back to our days of sharing ideas about medicine and health, where I was in awe of his vitality and presence. I learned, at that time, that his secret was his faithful adherence to a healthy lifestyle and meditation. With this work, Dr. Gutierrez continues to breathe life into age-old knowledge and highlight recent medical research findings. He confidently walks two worlds by highlighting the best in western medicine and the holistic aspect of yogic and Eastern philosophies. Whether you want to improve your health, want to solidify your health knowledge foundation, or be reminded of the important aspects of your life, let this book be your guiding light.

—Scott Mark Harrington, D.O.
Board Certified in Family Medicine
Creator of Dietnosis.com

The Daily Routine

Do you find yourself setting health goals for yourself year after year and not getting results? Are you frustrated because you seem to make the right health choices but are still not getting the results you desire? Do you have the knowledge but have difficulty putting it into practice to accomplish your health goals? Are you concerned about your health and want an all-natural lifestyle plan? Then this book is for you!

In this book, you will learn specific, scientifically proven principles of stress reduction. You will learn specific meditation and mindfulness techniques that will allow you to become proficient in controlling stress and creating your health destiny. Through the principles you will learn in this book, the subjective experience of time slows down, and you will experience more present-moment awareness. This state creates more willpower, awareness, and freedom to allow you to make the proper lifestyle choices for the long term. More importantly, this practice will engender long-term happiness and fulfillment. Once the mind, body, and emotions are balanced through proper nutrition, exercise, and meditation, you will experience vibrant health!

I wrote this book to share the secrets and scientifically proven principles I have been living in my personal life. I have also shared many of these principles with my patients during the past 12 years of practicing medicine. To my great delight, modern science is confirming that if you follow the principles in this book, you, too, can obtain superior health. I have divided this book into a simple format that will allow you to absorb the information quickly and put it into practice in your daily life. Each chapter begins with a story (or two), then an explanation of the principles and current scientific understanding of the concept for the intelligent reader. I close each chapter with take-home "Pearls." These "Pearls" at the end of each chapter function as a summary you can immediately implement in your daily life to reap the health benefits. The foundation of this entire book is based on our current scientific understanding of the practices conducive to health and longevity.

Planning is a crucial part of your success. Identify your long term goals, your vision, and your mission statement on a sheet of paper. Let's say you're depressed and fifty pounds overweight, you can write down, "I want to be happy and lose fifty pounds". This is your long-term goal. How will you get there? Through daily and weekly practice of the steps contained in this book. Once per week, plan out your entire week. Every evening plan out your meals, meditation, and exercise plan for the next day. Planning your daily routine is instrumental. You can use *The Daily Routine For Superior Health* companion workbook (free download at drorestesg.com).

I have had the privilege of learning the scientific practice of meditation under the guidance of world-renowned master teachers. I have been practicing and sharing these techniques for almost two decades. In the chapters that follow, I will delve deeply into the specific meditation and mindfulness techniques that will reduce stress and conquer emotional turbulence. Also, you will learn nutritional principles and develop an exercise plan that can reverse and prevent disease, thus attaining superior health.

Superior health is something that comes naturally to children. When you look at a child expressing joy, happiness, love, creativity, inquisitiveness, spontaneity, boundless energy, and a zest for life, realize that this is your natural inheritance! Movement and exercise comes easily and naturally for a child. They also naturally resonate with healthy foods like vegetables and fruits. Most children are free of mental stress; it is our natural state. Pain and hardships are universal, they exist in human life, regardless of race, gender, nationality, sexuality, or economic status. However, mental stress, worrying, and anxiety over events that one cannot control creates suffering. This type of mental worrying that creates suffering is unnecessary. There are universal teachings that give us a roadmap on how we can manage stress and avoid unnecessary suffering.

Part one begins with meditation and mindfulness training because it forms the cornerstone to superior health. Without deep roots in mindfulness, most health goals are fleeting or ill-advised. The restlessness mind runs wildly distracted on social media, being duped by endless unfounded claims by quacks on the internet, receiving misinformation from poorly qualified health educators and charlatans, and generally getting confused. Building a strong foundation in meditation and mindfulness will allow one to build sufficient willpower to follow through on your goals and have excellent physical, mental, and emotional health. I will teach you safe and effective principles that will allow you to follow a lifestyle plan conducive to excellent health. These lifestyle choices are made possible through controlling stress. This practice will allow you to stay focused on your health goals. By balancing the mind and keeping it peaceful and calm, your dreams and health destiny, which is superior health, will become reality!

Part One

Reducing Stress
through Mindfulness
and Meditation

CHAPTER ONE

REVERSE AGING
WITH STRESS REDUCTION

We must accept finite disappointment, but never lose infinite hope.
—MARTIN LUTHER KING, JR.

Because suffering is impermanent, that is why we can transform it.
Because happiness is impermanent, that is why we have to nourish it.
—THÍCH NHẤT HẠNH

DR. MARTIN LUTHER KING, JR. AND ZEN MASTER Thích Nhất Hanh were great friends. They both endured tremendous suffering and disappointments in their lives. Their strong faith and the practice of meditation and mindfulness allowed them to overcome enormous obstacles and transform suffering. Through this deep practice of meditation, they could reduce stress and never lose hope in their goals and dreams. They were both able to keep a peaceful and tranquil mind in the midst of external chaos and hardships. Therein lies the secret to superior health, the management and interpretation of subjective, perceived stress. Subjective, perceived stress is ephemeral and always illusory. However, its impact on the human mind and body are very real. Some common ways that this mental stress manifests is with symptoms of muscle tension, fatigue, depression, anxiety, insomnia, irritability, headache, anger outburst, addictions, emotional eating, social isolation, chest pain, tremors, heartburn, and skin diseases. In short, stress leads to chronic inflammation, depressed immune system, and hormone imbalance, which leads to disease and premature aging.[1,2] Let's delve deeper into the different types of stressors humans face and their detrimental health consequences. Then we will explore the tools, meditation and mindfulness, that help manage stress. That is the key to superior health.

In modern Western psychology and the ancient Eastern philosophy of Vedanta, there are three universal stressors that confront all humans. Cataclysmic stressors are natural disasters such as earthquakes, tsunamis, and hurricanes, and these events are uncontrollable and indeed lead to great pain. Then there are objective stressors. These include getting rear-ended in a car accident, a sprained ankle, or a fever. There's nothing you can do about those events. If you accidentally trip and fall and bruise your knee, this will cause pain and is an objective stressor that will afflict all humans. The last stressor that universally touches all humans is subjective mental stress. Subjective stress is perceived stress about all the things that are out of your control. The late Stephen Covey calls this worrying about your circle of concern, or the things you have no control over. Instead, focus on the circle of influence, or things you can directly control, like your attitude. Subjective, perceived mental stress, is avoidable and managed through a shift in perspective. It is therefore optional. Let's discuss recent research on how subjective stress impacts physical health.

How does our outer world affect our inner world? A paper published in 2004 investigated the effects of objective stress (environment-based) versus subjective stress (perception-based), in fifty-eight healthy premenopausal women.[3] The women were the biological mothers of either a healthy child or caregiver to chronically ill child. As expected, the women who were caregivers to chronically ill children had significantly higher stress levels. What is fascinating is that the authors found a significant correlation between high levels of perceived stress (subjective) and cellular aging, independent of care-giver status. In other words, your overall health is determined not so much by the circumstances in life, but by how your mind subjectively interprets your situation. Perceived stress has a tremendous impact on biological aging, and multiple studies corroborate these findings.

How can we use meditation to decrease our rate of biological aging? A recent study published in 2013 examined forty non-stressed with forty-one stressed subjects at work.[4] The study concluded that the hormone of youth, DHEA-S, was 23 percent lower in the subjects who reported stress at work compared to the non-stressed group. DHEA-S is produced by the adrenal cortex. Blood levels peak in the mid-twenties and there is a linear gradual decline with aging. Research shows that long-term meditators had a blood DHEA-S level that was comparable to someone up to 10 years younger.[5] Through meditation one can directly modulate biological aging by slowing down the age-related deterioration of DHEA-S through controlling stress.

Another major stress in people's everyday lives is work. A study published in 2012 examined 2,911 men and women, aged thirty to sixty-four, for work-related exhaustion.[6] After adjustment for age and sex, individuals with severe work-related exhaustion had an accelerated rate of biological aging as measured through leukocyte telomeres. It is fascinating to note that whether stress comes from work, being the primary care give to a sick child, or from worrying about the past or future, the effects on your physiology are profound.

These studies showing how chronic mental stress leads to premature aging confirm what I see in my clinical practice. Subjective stress (perceived), from my experience, leads to 75 percent of the problems that walk through my office door as a practicing physician. These patients with chronic stress look haggard. They have bags under their eyes from insomnia, excessive fat on the body from emotional eating and cortisol release, and excessive wrinkles and gray hairs. This stress can manifest in the physical body as muscle tension, headaches, fatigue, irritability, depressed immune system, crankiness, insomnia, impaired wound healing, acid reflux, stomach ache, forgetfulness, and anxiety. A stressed person's general appearance looks older than the stated chronological age. The biological age is usually older as well, with an elevated blood pressure, elevated blood sugar, and an elevated resting pulse. Furthermore, chronic stress affects psychological well-being and the patient usually does not have a healthy emotional expression, vibrancy, or overall happiness for being alive. Uncontrolled chronic stress directly impacts physical and mental well-being.

The first part of this book teaches techniques that you can start using today to reverse and even delay the effects of chronic stress. The cornerstone of any long-term health plan is deep relaxation through meditation. It is my professional opinion that, over time, patients tend to relapse because they lose focus of their health plan due to chronic uncontrolled stress. But what exactly is stress?

Modern psychology defines subjective or mental stress as an "emotional experience accompanied by predictable biochemical, physiological, and behavioral changes." Humans are hard-wired to respond to stress with the well-known fight or flight response, which is an unconscious reaction that happens in our autonomic nervous system. Without thinking, our sympathetic nervous system stimulates our adrenal glands to release stress hormones epinephrine and norepinephrine from the adrenal medulla. Emerging literature suggests humans actually have four responses to stress, namely fight, flight, freeze (to avoid detection by predators) or tend and befriend (usually a female response). In a cataclysmic event, such as an earthquake, it will of course, be natural and normal for your body to have physiological changes and release of stress hormones. However, in our society, in the midst of the hustle and bustle, one is releasing stress hormones in a traffic jam, in line at the grocery store, or at a business meeting at work. This chronic stress leads to disease. Research shows that chronic stress leads to premature aging by shortening telomeres and increasing oxidative stress. Unless the events are cataclysmic or objective (environment-based), then all other events are one's subjective interpretation of reality. This subjective experience of stress, which leads to unnecessary suffering, is our number one killer. Part one of this book will allow you to manage and interpret stress in a healthy way and avoid unnecessary pain and suffering that comes with chronic mental stress.

Approximately 25 percent of patients that walk through the door of my medical practice have chief complaints related to objective stress (environment-based), such as a rash, fever, whiplash from a car accident, sprained ankle, and back pain. When objective stressors happen, you fix them. A sprained ankle gets rest, ice, elevation, and anti-inflammatories. Lacerations get stitches, for example. Managing subjective stress is much more challenging. The best way for me to explain this important topic is to share a few momentous events in my life and how they relate to stress management. I hope to inspire the reader to know that any dream can become a reality with the help of stress reduction. I will also highlight how the daily practice of meditation and mindfulness has transformed my life from a stressed-out pre-med college student to a more centered and peaceful adult who is experiencing superior health. My journey was not easy.

As a four-year-old boy, I was uprooted from the communist country of Cuba as my parents searched for the American dream. A determined single mother of two raised me by working multiple jobs to pay the bills. As a young child, I focused on sports and gaining knowledge of the streets. All academics were neglected in pursuit of sports. It was my dream to play for Major League Baseball or the National Basketball Association.

In high school, my GPA and SAT scores were not good enough for college acceptance, so I enlisted in the Navy's dental hygienist program. As I prepared for boot camp, I received a momentous call from Dr. Rosa Jones from Florida International University. Dr. Jones told me that she ran a special program for minority students called the "Super Summer Program." If I showed that I could handle the college course work, I would be accepted into the fall semester. Needless to say, I was thrilled! I was the first person in my family to go to college!

As one can imagine, I entered college with great zest for learning and I was eager to transform my life. I felt that I had wasted twelve years of free education. With this newfound drive and passion for knowledge, I took on the daunting curriculum of pre-med with aspirations of becoming a doctor. As if a biology major with a premedical curriculum was not challenging enough, for some unfathomable reason I also decided to major in philosophy. So, as a double major pre-med student studying biology and philosophy, I earned 150 college credits and was on the Dean's list with a 3.5 GPA. However, I could not rest on my laurels. There was one final test standing between me and medical school.

The pressure of the Medical College Admissions Test (MCAT) was overwhelming. Knowing that my entire career hinged on one test was too much stress and pressure for me to handle at the time. The night before the MCAT, I tossed and turned all night and did not get even a wink of sleep. My restless mind was out of control. Thoughts were pouring endlessly from my mind, and my nervous system was on overdrive. The next morning during the test, I could not think straight or keep my eyes open. The sleepless night felt as if a truck had hit me, and I had no energy to function. All I could do was yawn and think about going to a warm bed. As you might imagine, I failed the biggest test of my life. I would not get into medical school and fulfill my dreams of becoming a doctor.

A radical change was necessary. During my summer break, I registered to retake the test and looked for a strategy to achieve different results. I delved deeply into the scientific practice of meditation and mindfulness training. Fortunately, there were world-renowned teachers that lived in Miami: Dr. Muata Ashby, Ph.D. and Swami Jyotirmayananda. I knew that it would help my nervous system relax and control my subjective stress. The science of meditation can lower blood pressure, reduce anxiety, lower heart rate, decrease stress, decrease inflammation, and modulate the immune system. Harvard researchers published a paper in 2013 showing how meditation can switch on and off some genes linked to stress and immune function.[7]

Even though there were scientific studies proving meditation can lower stress, there were also studies showing that most students don't improve much in standardized tests. In other words, there was not much hope for me to improve from my poor scores in the first MCAT. Perhaps I may have improved by one or two points, but that would not be enough for me to get into medical school. An enormous improvement was necessary.

The odds were stacked against me. Minority students with Spanish as their native language have a historically dismal performance on the MCAT.

Through the power of daily meditation and mindfulness, I slept like a baby the night before my second MCAT. My nervous system and mind were balanced, calm, and focused. With the weight of the world on my shoulders, I had a massive improvement on my second MCAT. Indeed, as a minority student with a 3.5 GPA, a double major, and a solid score on the MCAT, I got accepted to three medical schools. My dream of becoming a doctor was a reality!

Since 1998, I have continued a daily practice of meditation. I have found this scientific procedure to be one of the most effective methods to manage stress and help navigate me through obstacles in life. This practice has helped me in my personal relationships, work life, family life, creative endeavors, and in running. Not only has meditation helped me reduce the harmful effects of perceived stress, but it has shaped my attitude toward how I experience reality. It cannot be overstated that meditation and mindfulness slow down the rate of biological aging.[8] The key lies in how one interprets perceived stressors. The following story illustrates this point.

There is a parable that highlights how our perceived stress colors our experience of external reality and overall health: There were two men who lived in the same big city and were planning to relocate to a small town. The first man left the big city and was visiting the small town. A wise man stood at the entrance. He asked the wise man,

"How are the people in this commu
wise man replied, "How were the pe
old community?" The first man said,
were friendly, compassionate, trustworthy,
will miss them dearly." The wise man at the ʒ ᴊ
said, "That is exactly the type of people in this
community." The second traveler came to this
small town, and he asked the wise man the same
question. The wise man had the same response,
"How are the people in your old community?" The
second man replied, "Oh, they were highway rob-
bers, evil, mean, untrustworthy people." The wise
man said, "That is exactly the people you will find
in this community!"

The two men were given different answers to
the same question. This is because our subjective
experience of reality colors our experience of the
world. It is clear that our choice of attitude can
impact our perceived subjective stress, which in
turn will influence our physical health. Our perceived mental stress can manifest as muscle tension,
fatigue, headaches, decreased sex drive, anxiety,
depression, insomnia, restlessness, chest pain, upset
stomach, emotional eating, and addictions. In short,
subjective stress shapes how we see the world. Perceived stress is usually ephemeral and always illusory. However, its impact on the human mind and
body are very real and lead to disease. In the next
chapter we will learn practical steps of meditation
and mindfulness to help reduce and manage stress.

There are three types of universal stressors that humans face: cataclysmic stress (natural disasters), objective stress (environment-based), and subjective stress (perceived stress). Meditation and mindfulness will allow one to manage all three types of stressors in a healthy way. The secret to superior health is the management and interpretation of subjective stress. Subjective stress is usually ephemeral and always illusory. However, its impact on the human mind and body is very real and leads to disease. Realize that subjective (perceived) stress is influenced by your interpretation of reality. Subjective stress leads to premature aging and this can be prevented with a shift in awareness through mindfulness and meditation. No matter what cards you're dealt in life, through hard work and determination, anything is possible! Learn the art of meditation and mindfulness to help control stress and overcome obstacles in life. Once stress is controlled, the mind will be balanced, focused, and calm. A tranquil mind can handle any challenge life may present, and will allow you to formulate a health plan and follow through with it for the long term.

Chapter 1 Endnotes

1. Haigis MC, Yankner BA. The Aging Stress Response. *Molecular cell*. 2010;40(2):333-344. doi:10.1016/j. molcel.2010.10.002.

2. O'Donovan A, Slavich GM, Epel ES, Neylan TC. Exaggerated neurobiological sensitivity to threat as a mechanism linking anxiety with increased risk for diseases of aging. *Neuroscience and biobehavioral reviews*. 2013;37(1):96-108. doi:10.1016/j.neubiorev.2012.10.013.

3. Epel ES, Blackburn EH, Lin J, et al. Accelerated telomere shortening in response to life stress. *Proceedings of the National Academy of Sciences of the United States of America*. 2004;101(49):17312-17315. doi:10.1073/pnas.0407162101.

4. Lennartsson A-K, Theorell T, Rockwood AL, Kushnir MM, Jonsdottir IH. Perceived Stress at Work Is Associated with Lower Levels of DHEA-S. Esteban FJ, ed. *PLoS ONE*. 2013;8(8):e72460. doi:10.1371/journal.pone.0072460.

5. Glaser JL, Brind JL, Vogelman JH, et al. Elevated serum dehydroepiandrosterone sulfate levels in practitioners of the Transcendental Meditation (TM) and TM-Sidhi programs. *J Behav Med*. 1992;15(4): 327-341.

6. Ahola K, Sirén I, Kivimäki M, et al. Work-Related Exhaustion and Telomere Length: A Population-Based Study. Kiechl S, ed. *PLoS ONE*. 2012;7(7):e40186. doi:10.1371/journal.pone.0040186.

7. Bhasin MK, Dusek JA, Chang B-H, et al. Relaxation Response Induces Temporal Transcriptome Changes in Energy Metabolism, Insulin Secretion and Inflamma-

tory Pathways. Bai Y, ed. *PLoS ONE.* 2013;8(5):e62817. doi:10.1371/journal.pone.0062817.

8. Epel E, Daubenmier J, Moskowitz JT, Folkman S, Blackburn E. Can meditation slow rate of cellular aging? Cognitive stress, mindfulness, and telomeres. *Annals of the New York Academy of Sciences.* 2009;1172:34-53. doi:10.1111/j.1749-6632.2009.04414.x.

PRACTICAL STEPS FOR STRESS REDUCTION

*Do every act of your life as though it were the
very last act of your life.*

—MARCUS AURELIUS

*Meditation is all about the pursuit of nothingness. It's like the ulti-
mate rest. It's better than the best sleep you've ever had. It's a quieting
of the mind. It sharpens everything, especially your appreciation of
your surroundings. It keeps life fresh.*

—HUGH JACKMAN

*There are two ways to live: you can live as if nothing is a miracle; you
can live as if everything is a miracle.*

—ALBERT EINSTEIN

A FIFTY-SIX-YEAR-OLD PATIENT, MR. SMITH, HAD
suffered a traumatic event as a teenager. This traumatic event stayed with him for more than forty
years and still affects his life today. I shared with him
the teaching derived from *A Course in Miracles.*[1]
All present-moment events and situations can be
viewed as a choice between a grievance or a miracle.
The art is to choose the miracle. The present moment
has many conditions of joy and happiness available

to feel grateful for being alive. This present moment is a miracle. He continued to hold onto old emotional turbulence and anger toward his brother for the past 40 years. He could not forgive his brother but after hearing the exercise that I shared with him he decided to focus on the present moment and choose the miracle. Also, I reminded him of the saying, "When you forgive, you set a prisoner free. Then you realize the prisoner was you." My patient had the insight to release old grievances and choose the miracle. How did he have insight to do this? It requires space and the willpower to choose. This space and willpower is harnessed through the scientific practice of meditation.

Meditation and mindfulness increases one's willpower and freedom to choose. Most people live their lives in a very reactionary way. They walk around life aimlessly, letting external life circumstances determine their destiny. There is a stimulus (someone harshly criticizes you) and an immediate response (you angrily get defensive). Many times, this response comes without forethought. Of course, there are stimulus-response scenarios that are normal and physiologic, like the stimulus of a hot stove and the response of immediately moving the hand. What about the stimulus of a negative thought, past hurt, and emotional pain? Do these thoughts and feelings immediately trigger the response of smoking, drinking, or overeating to numb the pain? For a lot of people this is exactly what happens, and they are not even aware of it! There is no space between stimulus and response. Meditation and mindfulness create space and enlarge the conscious awareness between stimulus and response. With this space and heightened consciousness comes the freedom to choose your next action (response), and ideally you chose the miracle (positive). The next time that a negative thought, past hurt, or emotional pain comes, the secret is to become aware of it, and realize that those thoughts and feelings are not the real you. Then, transform those old grievances by choosing something positive in the miracle of the present moment. You can do something positive like exercising or reading, or just be with yourself and focus on the breath until the thoughts and feelings go away. This process is also known as the eternal witness. Stephen R. Covey said it well, "Between stimulus and response is our greatest power—the freedom to choose".

There is a very powerful quote by Dr. Victor Frankl in his classic book *Man's Search For Meaning*.[2] "Everything can be taken from a man but one thing: the last of the human freedoms—to choose one's attitude in any given set of circumstances, to choose one's own way." It is astonishing that Dr. Frankl chose to remain positive, even in the horrors of a Nazi concentration camp. His choice of attitude allowed him to survive.

The secret of mindfulness is to observe your thoughts and emotions as they surface and become aware of them in a nonjudgmental way. After a short while, you release them. They are not there to stay. You let them go, and they go away. A mnemonic device to help you remember the principle of witnessing any emotional turbulence when it surfaces is to think of the following: **HALT REAL Insight**. Each capital letter stands for a word to help you remember to observe your emotions and thoughts before reacting. This practice allows you the freedom to choose.

Hunger: Is hunger the source of your irritability and short fuse?

Anger: Are you angry and projecting your issues onto another person?

Lonely: Is loneliness causing you to overeat and create food addictions?

Tired: Are you tired, and this is leading to crankiness and poor health decisions?

Recognize: After you have observed the source of your emotions with HALT, if you are sad, just recognizing you are sad is the first step to healing.

Embrace: Once you recognize you are sad, angry, lonely, etc., you embrace this emotion and own up to this feeling.

Accept: Once you have recognized it and embraced it, you are no longer in denial, and you can accept it for what it is, a feeling or thought.

Look deeply: Once you have recognized it, embraced it, and accepted this emotion or thought, you can look deeply into its root cause.

Insight: Once you have gone through the procedure of **HALT REAL**, you will spontaneously have insight into yourself and feel better right away.

When my youngest son was almost ten years old, he was having trouble controlling his restless mind. He did not come out and directly tell me what was happening. In the fall of 2012, we were having a father-son moment. He became very sad. When I asked what was wrong, he immediately released lots of pent up emotions and many tears of sadness. With his lower lip trembling and his dimples conspicuously absent, he described what happened. He told me he recently read a book about monsters. He is very creative and imaginative, and this imaginary monster kept coming into his consciousness. Everywhere he looked, especially in the dark, but also during the day, he would see this monster from the book. He knew that this monster was not real, but his frustration and sadness was so immense that he could not control his thoughts. He asked me directly, "Dad, how can I control my thoughts?" while tears streamed down his face.

Immediately, I comforted my son, and told him it was all right to cry and express his emotions. Also, I let him know that everyone experiences moments of a restless mind. The key was to know that those thoughts are not real. Just observe them and let them go, I told him. I also wanted to share with him a scientifically proven technique to help control his mind. Synchronistically, I was drawn to the Bhagavad Gita, and I randomly opened to the page with the perfect lesson. I told my son that many, many years ago a great enlightened master shared with me this quotation from the Gita[3]:

> *If your mind is unsteady and wandering, many branched and endless are the thoughts and choices. When your mind is clear and one-pointed, there is only one decision.*

Just like the apprenticeship of heroes in movies like Star Wars, I told my son I had learned a secret ancient technique that has been passed down for thousands of years from teacher to student. He got excited about the training and practice when he heard about Jedi training. I taught him one of my favorite simple breathing meditation techniques. He was to practice this for one or two minutes in the morning and one or two minutes before going to bed. He started practicing this breathing meditation and immediately felt better.

Meditation is a universal tool that anyone can use to calm the mind and attain more peace. One can use meditation with their chosen religion. Meditation is a science developed by practitioners of yoga, Vedanta, and Buddhism thousands of years

ago. Yoga is a practice to help one attain enlightenment or liberation (moksha). Yoga is a Sanskrit term
that means "to unite." It helps unite the individual
with peace. Meditation is defined in *The Yoga Sutras
of Patanjali*[4] as follows:

> *3.1 Dharana is the binding of mind to
> one place, object or idea. 3.2 Dhyana is
> the continuous flow of cognition toward
> that object.*

The first step in the practice is to concentrate (be
mindful of an object). The concentration could
be on one's breath, a rose, an altar, a picture, a
candle, etc. In a calm and relaxed fashion, one
focuses all the attention on the object of concentration. If the mind wanders off to another thing
or thought, one gently brings it back to the object
of concentration. This training allows the mind to
spontaneously and effortlessly enter meditation.
In this state, the mind is alert, aware, calm, peaceful, and free of disturbances. With practice, this
state can be brought about in just a few seconds
through mindful breathing. As mentioned earlier,
the practice of meditation and mindfulness creates more space between stimulus and response in
one's day-to-day life. This ultimately creates more
freedom and allows one to create their own destiny.
It should be noted that meditation should not be
used only as a means to some end. Meditation and
mindfulness, with practice, are deeply rewarding

in and of themselves. The conscious awareness of your breath and the realization that you are alive in your body should bring immediate happiness. As Thich Nhất Hanh says, "The present moment is filled with joy and happiness. If you are attentive, you will see it."

The best time to have formal meditation practice is in the early morning hours. The Vedic sages identified the hours of 4:00-6:00 a.m. as being the best time for formal meditation practice since there is a special energy, peace, and stillness that heightens the experience during this time. If that time does not fit into your schedule, it's acceptable to meditate at any time in the morning. It is important, but not critical, to set up a sacred space in your home. Make a ritual dedicated to the practice of meditation so it will become a habit. The key is to meditate daily before embarking on your busy day. Marianne Williamson says it well, "Just as you wouldn't leave the house without taking a shower, you shouldn't start the day without at least ten minutes of sacred practice: prayer, meditation, inspirational reading."

If you can comfortably sit in the full lotus posture without pain in your body for meditation that is fantastic but not necessary. Sitting comfortably in a chair is acceptable. It is important to have an empty stomach. Wear appropriate clothing to keep the body comfortable. Use one of the formal meditation techniques discussed below for five to ten minutes, but you can go longer if you wish. Below are several of my favorite meditation exercises I have been practicing for many years.

Mindful Breathing Meditation

Sit quietly in a space with eyes open or closed. Keep a straight spine and observe the inflow and outflow of your breath. As you take a deep breath in, listen to your breath. As you breathe out, listen to your breath. Become aware of your thoughts as they come and let them go. When your mind gets lost in thoughts, bring it back to the awareness of your breath. That is all there is to this simple exercise of breath awareness that helps calm the restless mind and nervous system. There are hundreds of variations and modifications to the simple breathing meditation I described. I shall discuss variations that can be added to the simple breathing meditation.

So Hum Meditation

Continue with the mindful breathing meditation discussed above. As you breathe in, hear the sound "So" in your mind, and as you breathe out hear the sound "Hum" in your mind. This is the natural sound the breath makes when you breathe deeply and calmly. The practice is to breathe in and repeat "So" in your mind, and breathe out and repeat, "Hum" in your mind. Breathe in "So" and breathe out "Hum." So Hum is a sanskrit mantra meaning, "I am that." When you repeat the mantra "I am that," you remember that you are one with all of creation. It is a reminder that we are all interdependent with one another and everything in the cosmos.

Psalms 46:10 Meditation

Continue with the mindful breathing meditation discussed above. As you take in a deep breath, be aware of your breath, and as you breathe out, be aware of your breath. Become aware of your thoughts as they come and let them go. This time, synchronize your breathing with the mantra "Be still and know that I am God." As you breathe in, mentally repeat "Be still," and as you breathe out, mentally repeat "Know that I am God." Repeat this mantra from Psalms 46:10 for several minutes. Then, as you breathe in, mentally repeat "Be still," and as you breathe out, mentally repeat "Know that I am" for several minutes. Then, as you breathe in, mentally repeat "Be still," and as you breathe out mentally repeat "Know" for several minutes. Then, as you breathe in, mentally repeat "Be," and as you breathe out, mentally repeat "Still" for several minutes. Lastly, take a deep relaxing breath in and mentally repeat "Be," and let out a deep relaxing breath slowly while mentally repeating "Be," breathing in "Be" and breathing out "Be." Continue with this meditation for several minutes. I learned this beautiful meditation from the late Swami Satchitananda while visiting his ashram in Yogaville.

Vedanta Wisdom Meditation

Sit quietly in a space with eyes open or closed. Keep a straight spine and observe the inflow and outflow of the breath. As you take a deep breath in, be aware of your breath, and as you breathe out, be aware of your breath. Become aware of your thoughts as they come and let them go. With a peaceful and calm mind silently repeat to yourself the phrase: "Nothing exists. Nothing belongs to me. I am neither mind nor body. Immortal self am I." Continue repeating this ancient mystic song several times. Feel the profundity and the truth of these words. I learned this profound lesson from Swami Jyotirmayananda. I use this meditation while running sometimes and especially during races. It is a great sports psychology tool to endure pain in a race.

True Home Meditation

Continue with breath awareness. As you breathe in, repeat "I have arrived" in your mind, and as you breathe out, repeat "I am home" in your mind. This will naturally bring you back to the present moment. As you breathe in, stay mindful of your breath and know "I have arrived" and breathe out and know "I am home." The full mantra is breathing in "I have arrived," breathing out "I am home," breathing in "in the here," breathing out "in the now." I learned this beautiful mantra from the Zen Master Thich Nhất Hanh. It immediately brings the mind back to the body and engenders present-moment awareness.

This meditation brings you back to your true home address, which is always the Here and the Now.

Grace at Dinner Meditation

One practice I do regularly with my family is saying grace at the dinner table. We look gratefully at our food and give thanks to it. We go around the table and everyone has a turn saying what they are thankful for on the plate. Everyone at the table gives thanks to a particular item on the plate and visualizes where that food comes from. For example, if we are eating guacamole, the kids would thank the avocado tree and the sun that helps it grow. In the tofu stir fry, someone would give thanks to the soybean and visualize how the soybean plant looks and where it grows. Once we run out of food items to thank, we thank the farmers for growing our food, and then we thank the cook, etc. In this fashion, we feel an appreciation for how our food gets on our table and we feel interconnected with each other and all of creation.

One effective way to engender a feeling of gratitude in one's daily life is to ask the following questions at the end of each day. What surprised you? What moved you? What inspired you? What made you laugh? What enriched you? If one faces life with this attitude, it will certainly engender more gratitude and a smile. In every situation, one can focus on scarcity or abundance. This exercise will allow one to choose abundance.

Informal Meditation Practice

This is the practice of living every moment of one's life mindfully in the present moment. This is different from the formal practice of "sit down" meditation. This practice is done while walking, talking, eating, or doing any of the myriad of things in daily life. It involves being aware of the present moment and accepting it in a nonjudgmental way. One of the best ways to practice being present in the "now" is by doing breathing meditation. The practitioner is aware of his or her thoughts, emotions, and situations as they arise in one's daily life, and the practitioner anchors themselves in the present moment with deep mindful breathing. Mindfulness is being aware of the present moment in a nonjudgmental way and giving 100 percent of your attention to the "now."

PEARLS FROM CHAPTER 2

Create a formal meditation practice of ten to twenty minutes daily. This sacred time is the highest form of self-care. It should be a daily ritual. This quiet time is food for the soul and is a powerful adjunct to any religion. More importantly, practice informal meditation (mindfulness) throughout the day. Choose the meditation technique that is comfortable and comes naturally. The secret is a daily consistent practice of formal ("sit down") and informal ("mindfulness throughout the day") meditation.

This practice will allow the mind to stay calm and focused throughout the day on the goals and dreams you have for yourself. Mindfulness throughout the day is instrumental. Objectively observe turbulent emotions with the "HALT REAL Insight" witnessing technique. The practice of meditation and mindfulness creates more space between stimulus and response in one's day-to-day life. This ultimately creates more freedom to choose the truth and allows one to create their own destiny.

Chapter 2 Endnotes

1. Schucman H. *A Course in Miracles.* 2nd ed. New York, NY: Viking Press;1996.

2. Frankl, VE. *Man's Search for Meaning.* 1st ed. Boston, MA: Beacon Press;2006.

3. Saraswati, Sri Swami Satchidananda (1988). *The Living Gita: The Complete Bhagavad Gita - A Commentary for Modern Readers.* Yogaville: Integral Yoga Publications.

4. Saraswati, Sri Swami Satchidananda (2012). *Yoga Sutras of Patanjali,* Yogaville: Integral Yoga Publications.

CHAPTER THREE

HEALTH BENEFITS OF MEDITATION AND MINDFULNESS

The mind can go in a thousand directions, but on this beautiful path, I walk in peace. With each step, the wind blows. With each step, a flower blooms.

—THÍCH NHẤT HẠNH

Meditation is the dissolution of thoughts in Eternal awareness or Pure consciousness without objectification, knowing without thinking, merging finitude in infinity.

—VOLTAIRE

THE CORNERSTONE OF ANY LONG-TERM HEALTH plan is deep relaxation through meditation. It is my professional opinion that, over time, patients tend to relapse because they lose focus of their health plan due to chronic uncontrolled stress. Superior health is dependent on having a controlled response to stressors, achievable through a mindfulness practice.

Mrs. Davis is a thirty-nine-year-old executive who presented herself to my clinic with a chief complaint of fatigue, weight loss, and a ravenous appetite. She did not understand how she could be eating so much and still losing weight. When I checked her blood work, hemoglobin A1C was 11.7. This is a number used to diagnose diabetes. Over the past three months, her blood sugar was extremely elevated, averaging close to 300. A normal blood sugar average over three months should be closer to 100. She was a high level executive with a very stressful job requiring a busy travel schedule. The nature of her job caused her to be wired, always on the go, and eating fast food on the run. Many years of job stress and poor health choices led to a new diagnosis of diabetes mellitus.

I taught her a mindful breathing meditation technique that would allow her to control her stress levels and make wise health choices. We partnered in developing a health plan that included this meditation, and in just three months her A1C was less than 6.0. While we had discussed nutrition in the past, it was not until Mrs. Davis could control and manage her stress well with meditation that she could comply with her treatment plan. Furthermore, this allowed her to read literature on how to reverse her diabetes. Currently I am working with this patient on slowly weaning her from her medication and controlling her diabetes strictly through diet and exercise.

The vast majority of patient visits to their primary care doctor can be attributed to stress. Missed work and lessened productivity due to illness from chronic stress costs U.S. companies $300 billion a year, according to World Health Organization estimates.[1] Here is a trivia question I ask medical students: "What is directly or indirectly the cause of every human disease? This one thing could be linked to cancer, heart disease, diabetes, hypertension, alcoholism, drug abuse and overdoses, obesity, smoking, etc." The answer is stress. Specifically, chronic stress.

In contrast, the human nervous system is exquisitely designed to handle acute stress. Our nervous system has the "fight or flight" response that in a matter of seconds prepares us to fight the proverbial sabertooth tiger or run away from it. Faced with danger, our adrenal glands increase the production of cortisol, norepinephrine, epinephrine, and decrease nitric oxide. These stress hormones cause our body to increase oxygen consumption, increase blood pressure, increase heart rate, and divert blood to our muscles to run or fight. This increase in sympathetic nervous system stimulation was a great way to avoid the dangers when humans lived in the jungle and dealt with the threat of wild animals. The problem we face today is that most people activate this life or death stress response over the most trivial non-urgent things.

In modern, industrialized society, most of us don't have to worry about being attacked by wild animals. However, most of the stimulation to our "fight or flight" in our society comes from daily traffic jams, work burnout, email in-boxes, to-do lists, violent television, and violent music. This constant daily stimulation of our sympathetic nervous system leads to chronic stress and the detrimental downstream effects. This can lead to increased blood sugar, increased fat accumulation, protein breakdown, and a weakened immune system. Over time, chronic stress can lead to autoimmune diseases, cancer, cardiovascular disease, insomnia, fatigue, and increased infections and psychiatric diseases.

The great news is that there is a simple procedure that anyone can perform to immediately reduce stress. Our nervous system also has the opposite of the "fight or flight" response that is known as the "rest and digest." In this state, we have a decrease in stress hormones such as cortisol, epinephrine, norepinephrine, and increased nitric oxide. When our parasympathetic nervous system is stimulated, we have a lower heart rate, lower blood pressure and decreased oxygen consumption. The scientific procedure of meditation will produce a calm mind and a relaxed body and allow us to make excellent health choices.

The Harvard Professor Herbert Benson, M.D., coined the term "relaxation response" in the 1970s.[2] This happens when we voluntarily tap into or activate our parasympathetic nervous system. The good news is that you do not have to be an advanced practitioner of meditation to reap the benefits. Dr. Benson has shown that even novice practitioners can reap immediate benefits from one session of relaxation-response. Through one session of meditation, a practitioner can alter gene expression that is associated with stress and inflammation. Dr. Benson's research showed that long-term meditators had 2,000 stress-reducing genes activated compared to those who do not meditate. The great news is that once novices learned to meditate for twenty minutes per day for eight weeks, they had activated 1,500 genes associated with stress reduction![3] A study published in 2015 using biosensors to measure physiologic changes in both novice and experienced meditators found beneficial changes in brainwaves and blood pressure in both groups.[4]

It is not surprising that more and more studies are coming out showing a positive link between meditation and reduction in the aging process as measured by telomerase activity. These results indicate that chronic stress leads to premature aging at the cellular level. Also, chronic stress leads directly or indirectly to many chronic diseases that are associated with premature aging and an early death. There is exciting new research showing the effects of meditation on neuroplasticity and how meditation is a form of exercise for the brain.

How difficult is it to reap the benefits of meditation? Do you have to move to the Himalayan mountains for a nine-month silent retreat and meditate in the lotus posture for eight hours a day to reap the benefits of neuroplasticity? The answer is *no*.

Let's explore a recent study. Harvard neuroscientist Dr. Sara Lazar studied sixteen participants, and after eight weeks, meditation strengthened many regions of the brain. Specifically this study showed that the brain regions that strengthened were the hippocampus, cingulate cortex, temporoparietal junction, and cerebellum.[5] The old adage, "If you don't use it, you lose it" also applies to the brain, and this study shows the meditators literally have bigger brains. The participants in this study were meditation-naive and used Mindfulness-Based Stress Reduction (MBSR) as taught by Jon Kabat-Zinn, Ph.D. MBSR involves eight weekly group meetings and formal mindfulness training exercises. Mindfulness is defined as awareness of present-moment experiences with a compassionate, non-judgmental stance. Each day, the participants listened to a forty-five-minute audio recording that guided them through body scan, yoga, and sitting meditation. The results suggest that MBSR can positively affect brain regions involved in learning, memory, emotional regulation, self-referential processing, and perspective taking.

The brain is a fascinating organ. Your brain has 100 billion neurons and 100 trillion connections. Although neuroplasticity is an exciting new field in neuroscience, the yogis have been talking about transforming the mind and body through the power of meditation for centuries. The late Paramahansa Yogananda was discussing the power of meditation to transform the brain almost 100 years ago before the advent of functional MRI testing. In fact, the 2014 documentary *Awake: The Life of Yogananda* asserts that the yogi was discussing the process of neuroplasticity some 100 years before it was coined.

Furthermore, we know that Mahatma Gandhi was a yoga practitioner and practiced meditation daily. Specifically, we know that meditation can help strengthen the brain centers related to compassion. Nowadays we can measure precisely the effects of different types of meditation techniques on different brain centers.

In America, one in five people take a psychiatric medication. We spend more than 15 billion on psychiatric drugs and billions more on mental health care. Meditation is a safe and effective modality that can help the mental health crisis in this country. A paper published in 2013 compared twenty-five long term meditators with novices. This study used a different type of meditation technique known as Loving-Kindness meditation.[6] Compared to novices, the Loving-Kindness meditation experts had more gray matter volume detected in the right angular and posterior parahippocampal gyri as measured by 3T magnetic resonance imaging scanner. These regions are important for empathy, anxiety, and mood regulation. Furthermore, meta-analysis published in *JAMA Internal Medicine* in March 2014 found some compelling evidence for the use of meditation for dimensions of psychological stress.[7]

The study concluded that there is evidence for mindfulness meditation improving anxiety, depression, pain, and mental health–related quality of life. This is exciting research! Meditation is a powerful tool you can perform at any time, anywhere, with no negative side effects. Imagine the benefits of teaching daily meditation practice in the school systems in America.

Another health crisis happening in America is the overdiagnosis and overtreatment of attention deficit disorder. There are studies in Europe showing that attention deficit disorder is more of a product of social environment and parenting techniques than a pathology of the child's brain per se. For example, in the United States 9 percent of school-age kids have a diagnosis of ADHD and take pharmaceuticals, whereas in France less than 0.5 percent have the diagnosis. The paradigm is different since in France they look for an underlying cause in the social context and in America we view it as a pathological biological process. What can we do to help a growing brain? A recent study explored how several meditation techniques affect the brain in terms of concentration. Researchers used concentration, Loving-Kindness, and Choiceless Awareness meditation practices to see how they impact mind-wandering, which is the default mode for humans.[8] The premise is that mind-wandering correlates with unhappiness and that living in the present moment increases happiness. The researchers found that all three types of meditation techniques decreased mind-wandering both at baseline and during meditation. If parents learned simple meditation techniques to help increase happiness and help decrease mind wandering, it is my professional opinion that there would be fewer diagnoses of attention deficit disorder. Also, parents can teach their children a simple breathing meditation technique that can be performed for one to two minutes every day that will help tremendously.

Another concern in American healthcare is the overuse of narcotic painkillers. An estimated 2 million people abused prescription painkillers in 2013, according to the Center for Disease Control. Every year more people die from drug overdoses than from from motor vehicle collisions. Chronic pain can be a problem but there are promising ways to help treat chronic pain that do not involve the toxic and potentially life-threatening side effects of taking a painkiller. Meditation also has implication for the treatment of chronic pain. Recent studies have shown that meditators have increased brain size as shown via functional MRI. A study by Dr. Joshua Grant and colleagues published in 2010 studied seventeen meditators with eighteen controls.[9] Meditators had significantly lower pain sensitivity which was associated with having a thicker cortex in the anterior cingulate and in the somatosensory cortex. Instead of going directly to a dangerous and potentially deadly narcotic drug to treat pain, physicians should consider the safer modality of meditation to treat chronic pain.

Reducing stress is one of the most important things an individual can do for overall health and especially heart health. Everyday in the the United States 2,200 people die of cardiovascular disease. Health care expenditures are $312.6 billion annually for the treatment of heart disease and stroke. It has been known for decades there are higher incidences of heart attacks and strokes on Monday more than any other day of the week. Why? It is postulated that the stress hormones released in preparing for the work week increase blood pressure, arrhythmias, and inflammation. What can be done about this? Meditate every day and especially on weekends when one has more free time in preparation for the week. Meditation has shown to be beneficial to the body by strengthening the brain regions to help combat stress, decreasing C-reactive protein, improving perception and neural response to pain, improving immune function, and lowering blood pressure.

There are countless studies showing that meditation can positively affect neuroplasticity. Meditation can give you a stronger and bigger brain better able to handle stress. Stress will always be the universal presence in human life. The question is how will one interpret it and process it. By practicing meditation, we can deal with life stress in a more effective way. There will always be a dance between pain and joy in life. Meditation allows us to handle both artistically.

In Dr. Joseph Campbell's work, he notes that life has equal parts pain and pleasure, tragedy and comedy.[10] The great philosophers from ancient times observed a continuum of pleasure and pain. Similarly, Dr. Campbell has observed in mythologies throughout history a continuum of tragedy and comedy, the yin and yang, a game of hide and seek. In Vedic thought, it is Maya, the cosmic play, the magic show of the universe.

The experience of childbirth illustrates this point. Childbirth is a very painful experience. However, from this pain an enormous joy is produced from the birth of a new baby. Similarly, a delicious food can produce great joy. However, eating too much of this food can produce the pain of addiction. Indeed, Dr. Campbell states, "We cannot cure the world of sorrow, but we can choose to live in joy."

Meditation and mindfulness allow us to interpret and manage the pain and stress of life in a healthy way and give us the freedom to choose joy.

The first aspect of meditation is to stop. Stop the running here and there, day and night. After stopping, the practitioner calms the mind through mindful breathing meditation, allowing the mind and body to rest and heal. This whole process can take just a few minutes. The direct result of this practice is that stress hormones are reduced and the rate of aging slows.[11] The indirect result is that when confronted with a stimulus that, in the past, would have led to sadness and overeating, the practitioner now becomes aware and witnesses the emotions without mindlessly reacting. It is important to note that emotional turbulence can involve the restlessness that comes from excitement, happiness, agitation, and sadness, etc., which can take away mental peace and emotional equanimity.

Remember the mnemonic device discussed in Chapter Two, HALT REAL Insight, which can be used to objectively witness emotions and thoughts without reacting. This is the secret of your day-to-day informal meditation practice. This is mindfulness of the present moment. The procedure is very simple but profound. You observe your thoughts and emotions as they surface and become aware of them in a nonjudgmental way. After a short while, you release them. They are not there to stay; you let them go and they go away. Use the mnemonic device to help you remember the principle of witnessing negative emotions or thoughts when they surface: HALT REAL Insight. Refer to Chapter Two for the meaning of each letter.

As an example, imagine you are a traveler on the train carrying a heavy backpack. You get on the train and remain standing with an extremely heavy backpack. The train picks up speed, and it's going seventy-five mph, and it will arrive at its destination in twenty-four hours. But as the train is traveling, you are still standing and holding on to your heavy backpack. A wise man who is sitting in the train looks at you and says, "Why don't you take off that heavy backpack and sit down. Have a seat and enjoy the journey!" This story is an analogy for the unnecessary suffering that humans put themselves through. Life is always filled with heavy backpacks. The key is to learn to put down the heavy burden of the backpack. Let the train carry your heavy load and guide you to your next destination. Let go of stress and enjoy the journey.

PEARLS FROM CHAPTER 3

Chronic stress directly or indirectly leads to most modern diseases in industrialized societies. Meditation decreases stress hormones such as cortisol, epinephrine, and norepinephrine. This leads to lower heart rate, lower blood pressure, and decreased oxygen consumption. Through the practice of meditation one can decrease stress hormones, reduce anxiety, decrease inflammation, increase neuroplasticity, improve the immune system, and slow the aging process. Mindfulness allows one to live in the present moment thereby increasing happiness. Meditation and mindfulness allow us to interpret and manage the stress of life in a healthy way and give us the freedom to choose joy, and engender health.

CHAPTER 3 ENDNOTES

1. JP Brun. Work-related stress: scientific evidence-base of risk factors, prevention and costs. World Health Organi-

zation Stress at the Workplace. 2006. http://www.who.int/occupational_health/topics/brunpres0307.pdf

2. Benson H. *The Relaxation Response*. New York, NY: HarperCollins; 2000.

3. Bhasin MK, Dusek JA, Chang B-H, et al. Relaxation Response Induces Temporal Transcriptome Changes in Energy Metabolism, Insulin Secretion and Inflammatory Pathways. Bai Y, ed. *PLoS ONE*. 2013;8(5):e62817. doi:10.1371/journal.pone.0062817.

4. Steinhubl SR, Wineinger NE, Patel S, et al. Cardiovascular and nervous system changes during meditation. *Frontiers in Human Neuroscience*. 2015;9:145. doi:10.3389/fnhum.2015.00145.

5. Hölzel BK, Carmody J, Vangel M, et al. Mindfulness practice leads to increases in regional brain gray matter density. *Psychiatry research*. 2011;191(1):36-43. doi:10.1016/j.pscychresns.2010.08.006.

6. Brewer JA, Worhunsky PD, Gray JR, Tang Y-Y, Weber J, Kober H. Meditation experience is associated with differences in default mode network activity and connectivity. *Proceedings of the National Academy of Sciences of the United States of America*. 2011;108(50):20254-20259. doi:10.1073/pnas.1112029108.

7. Goyal M, Singh S, Sibinga EMS, et al. Meditation Programs for Psychological Stress and Well-being: A Systematic Review and Meta-analysis. *JAMA internal medicine*. 2014;174(3):357-368. doi:10.1001/jamainternmed.2013.13018.

8. Leung M-K, Chan CCH, Yin J, Lee C-F, So K-F, Lee TMC. Increased gray matter volume in the right angular

and posterior parahippocampal gyri in loving-kindness meditators. *Social Cognitive and Affective Neuroscience.* 2013;8(1):34-39. doi:10.1093/scan/nss076.

9. Grant JA1, Courtemanche J, Duerden EG, Duncan GH, Rainville P. Cortical thickness and pain sensitivity in zen meditators. *Emotion.* 2010 Feb;10(1):43-53. doi: 10.1037/a0018334.

10. Campbell J. *The Power of Myth.* New York, NY: Anchor; 1991.

11. Epel E, Daubenmier J, Moskowitz JT, Folkman S, Blackburn E. Can meditation slow rate of cellular aging? Cognitive stress, mindfulness, and telomeres. *Annals of the New York Academy of Sciences.* 2009;1172:34-53. doi:10.1111/j.1749-6632.2009.04414.x.

Part Two

Nutritional Excellence for Disease Prevention and Reversal

CHAPTER FOUR

Mindful Eating for Weight Loss

So often, even when we stop to say a blessing before a meal, we're mentally preparing to spoon some pasta or potatoes onto our plates. We're not usually focused on the present moment, simply placing ourselves before our food and entering into the still, slow space where eating is done for eating's sake and not something we do simply to get to the next thing on our list.

—Mary DeTurris Poust, *Cravings: A Catholic Wrestles with Food, Self-Image, and God*

Food for the body is not enough. There must be food for the soul.

—Dorothy Day

We are not human beings on a spiritual journey. We are spiritual beings on a human journey.

—Stephen R. Covey

And Jesus answered him, saying, "It is written, that man shall not live by bread alone, but by every word of God."

—Luke 4:4

A patient of mine is a forty-eight year old male who was fifty-seven pounds overweight. He would always eat on the run while in the car or standing in the kitchen. Habitually, he sedated himself by snacking late into the night. I shared with him a mindful breathing practice to engender present moment awareness. Also, I gave him strict rules of only eating when he could be fully present, sitting down at the table without distractions. With this practicing of mindful eating he has lost thirty pounds and is feeling much better.

Humans need three types of food to be healthy. Food for the body, mind, and soul. If we don't feed our mind and soul the proper foods, it is my experience that people will resort to toxic foods for the body. In today's society, people are constantly bombarded with information from commercials, family, friends, pyramid schemes, web pages, radio, and endless sources of "expert opinion." People are brainwashed by the "tribe," or the cultural influences and peer pressure from the masses. This influence is so powerful that people will do unhealthy things such as smoke tobacco, drink alcohol to excess, and eat the unhealthy Standard American Diet if that is what everyone else is doing. According to the author of *The Four Agreements*, Don Miguel Ruiz, this process is known as the domestication of humans, and you lose your freedom. Caroline Myss states it well: "The tribal mentality effectively indoctrinates an individual into the tribe's beliefs, ensuring that all believe the same." It takes strong conviction and strong willpower to be in the minority and directly go against what the masses of society are doing. If we honor and respect ourselves, we will not be tempted to resort to extreme measures to alter our bodies.

It is fascinating to note the extreme measures that humans will take to attain their ideal body weight. The human species has resorted to toxic starvation diets, dangerous supplements, surgeries, and even eating a tapeworm for weight-loss. Among fad supplements, we have seen 2,4-dinitrophenol, ephedra, hydroxycut, fen-phen, excessive caffein-ated beverages or pills, herbal xenicol, phentermine, and Meridia just to name a few.[1] These supplements can lead to death. Although most have been banned, they continue to be abused in the black market. If taking a pill that could lead to death sounds too risky, examine gastric bypass surgery. The risks of gastric bypass surgery include infection, blood clots, bleeding, bowel obstruction, leaks, dumping syndrome, gallstones, hernia, stomach perfora-tion, ulcers, and death. But the most dreaded risk of all, is going through this risky surgery and then having the stomach stretch out again and enlarge as the person re-gains the weight. Unfortunately, this happens to a significant percentage of patients who have this surgery. The FDA approved a safer alternative recently.

The ORBERA is a saline filled balloon inserted in the stomach using a minimally invasive endo-scopic procedure. The patient must be obese with a body mass index of 30-40 kg/m^2, have an obesity-related condition such as diabetes, hypertension, or hyperlipidemia, and have been unsuccessful in losing weight through diet and exercise. Studies are promising and patients using ORBERA on average lost twenty-two pounds after six months. This new procedure is not without its risks and possible side effects include gastric ulcers, indigestion, abdominal pain, vomiting, infection, allergic reaction, and rarely myocardial infarction. I would recommend ORBERA over gastric bypass surgery. However, I recommend mindful eating as a first-line therapy.

Americans are habituated to a materialistic lifestyle and are always on the go. There is a restless energy of constant doing and constant going. This constant running around is what makes people in modern industrialized societies feel alive. The fuel or food that keeps people running is material excess and overconsumption of things. This causes unnecessary mental stress. There is never dedicated time for being and nourishing the soul. Multitasking has become the norm. Eastern wisdom recommends the practice of stopping. Once you stop, the next step is calming. This practice of stopping and calming allows for resting and healing. Nowadays, even the sacred act of eating is undermined by discussing the "things to do" in a business meeting, or going to a noisy restaurant and watching a band play, or any of the myriad distractions we have while eating. There is nothing inherently wrong with these activities; it is just that in America it has become the norm. This constant restlessness on external distractions instead of focusing on digestion can lead to the overconsumption of food. Ignoring the body's satiety center and signals to stop eating is a crime against the wisdom of millions of years of built in evolution. Our body orchestrates and synchronizes countless chemical reactions and releases hormones to help us assimilate our food. For example, the stomach and small intestine release ghrelin, the "hunger hormone," which helps regulate appetite. Once the stomach is stretched, the secretion of ghrelin stops. Obesity and overeating negatively impact this important hormone ghrelin that is associated with satiety, hedonic eating, metabolic and cardiovascular health, and is anti-aging.[2] When we lose touch with these natural bodily signals, it leads to a slippery slope of overconsumption and disease. Distractions, or not eating mindfully, lead to not only overeating foods, but also to eating the wrong foods.

Hari Hachi bu is a Confucian teaching that means "eat only until you are 80 percent full." Also, in Ayurveda, it is taught to eat the equivalent of your two hands opened in the shape of a bowl or offering. This teaching is known as 'anjali'. These ancient mindfulness principles can remind us we must honor natural body signals to keep a healthy temple (body). This practice is used regularly by the Okinawan elders and is thought to contribute to their exceptional longevity.[3] Okinawans have the highest rate of centenarian per 100,000 people in the population, and this relative calorie restriction plays a role. They also have a very healthy body mass index (BMI).

A review article published in 2014 shows evidence for mindfulness-based intervention for obesity-related eating behaviors such as emotional eating.[4] Mindful eating creates lightness and freedom to choose to feel good by not overeating. Being mindful of consumption can be as simple as the ancient saying "eat when you are hungry and drink when you are thirsty." What may lead humans to overconsumption of food, and especially unhealthy foods, is determined by stress. A recent study suggests that stress may compromise self-control. Researchers examined the effects of acute stress on self-control and how this affects the brain.[5] Investigators noted that stress impairs self-control and affects brain regions such as the amygdala, striatum, and prefrontal cortex. The participants who were under stress in the study chose unhealthy foods although they had intentions of eating healthy. Stress in daily life and loss of self-control while eating has become the norm in our society.

In some Eastern traditions they take eating mindfully to a whole new level. In the dining hall, there can be hundreds of monks eating their meals in complete silence. In this way, they are honoring the food. Eating in this fashion is a form of meditation. The digestive fire, referred to as agni in Ayurveda, is fully focused on assimilating the nutrition entering the body.

My personal practice is to visualize the food in nature. If I am eating an apple, I see the apple tree basking in the Northwest sun, the cool breeze shaking the leaves, and the rain nourishing its roots. With each bite, I honor the interconnectedness of nature and all the elements and forces that allowed this wonderful fruit to sustain my body.

If I am at home with my family, this practice extends to the Grace at Dinner meditation described in Chapter Two.

When we eat mindfully, we see we are all inter-connected. We respect and honor all life on earth, including our pets. Let us take mindful eating to a whole new level by bringing this mindfulness to our beloved companion animals.

In America, we view eating dog meat as taboo and we protect our dogs, for they are man's best friend. However, did you know that even in America, it is legal in forty-four states to humanely kill one's dog and eat the dog meat for personal consumption? It is illegal to sell dog meat or serve it in restaurants in all fifty states. Does anyone reading this book view puppies as a delicacy? How about a baby calf or veal? I would make a strong argument that eating dog meat or cow meat is equally harm-ful for the human body. Furthermore, if you find it acceptable to eat cow's meat but not acceptable to eat dog's meat, that is speciesist. Speciesism is discrimination against animals. Discrimination is the highest form of arrogance. Anyone can be speciesist and discriminate against animals, irrespective of religious affiliation. For example, an atheist can say that humans are at the top of the food chain and use "survival of the fittest" as reasons we could eat dog meat. A religious person may say "God gave us dominion over all animals" as a reason to eat cow meat. At their core, all world religions teach peace, love, and being good stewards of the earth. If one looks deeply into cow meat and dog meat, we realize they are both the same. Both the cow and the dog have the right to exist, be free and be happy.

Mindful eating involves a shift in consciousness. It involves a realization that we are all one big family. Modern science tells us all life on earth is interconnected. When we honor the planet, we only consume the blessings given to us and avoid over-consumption. Controlling stress is important, so one's self-control in choosing the right foods is not sabotaged. If we only consume what our body desires, from true hunger, we will naturally and effortlessly attain our ideal body weight.[6] Research shows stress reduction and mindfulness can facilitate weight loss.[7,8] If you eat mindfully and you are currently at your ideal weight, you will maintain it. If you are not at your ideal weight and start eating mindfully, you will lose weight and attain your ideal weight spontaneously. The secret to a regular mindful eating practice is stress reduction.

Pearls from Chapter 4

Eating is a sacred act of connecting to the life force and energy of our universe through earth, wind, sun, and rain. Eat slowly in a mindful way and remember the ancient wisdom of hara hachi bu (stop eating once your stomach is 80 percent full). Only eat an anjali, the portion size of your two hands cupped in the shape of a bowl. Eat only when you feel hunger signals from your body. If you mindfully eat only what your body desires, you will naturally and effortlessly attain your ideal body weight. When we honor the planet we only consume healthy plant food that the body needs and avoid overconsumption. Controlling stress is crucial, so we can have the forethought to practice mindful eating every day.

Chapter 4 Endnotes

1. Grundlingh J, Dargan PI, El-Zanfaly M, Wood DM. 2,4-Dinitrophenol (DNP): A Weight Loss Agent with Significant Acute Toxicity and Risk of Death. *Journal of Medical Toxicology.* 2011;7(3):205-212. doi:10.1007/s13181-011-0162-6.

2. Buss J, Havel PJ, Epel E, Lin J, Blackburn E, Daubenmier J. Associations of ghrelin with eating behaviors, stress, metabolic factors, and telomere length among overweight and obese women: Preliminary evidence of attenuated ghrelin effects in obesity? *Appetite.* 2014;76:84-94. doi:10.1016/j.appet.2014.01.011.

3. Willcox BJ, Willcox DC, Todoriki H, et al. Caloric restric-

tion, the traditional Okinawan diet, and healthy aging: the diet of the world's longest-lived people and its potential impact on morbidity and life span. *Ann NY Acad Sci.* 2007;1114:434-455.

4. O'Reilly GA, Cook L, Spruijt-Metz D, Black DS. Mindfulness-Based Interventions for Obesity-Related Eating Behaviors: A Literature Review. *Obesity reviews : an official journal of the International Association for the Study of Obesity.* 2014;15(6):453-461. doi:10.1111/obr.12156.

5. Maier SU, Makwana AB, Hare TA. Acute Stress Impairs Self-Control in Goal-Directed Choice by Altering Multiple Functional Connections within the Brain's Decision Circuits. *Neuron.* 2015;87(3):621-631.

6. Fuhrman J, Sarter B, Glaser D, Acocella S. Changing perceptions of hunger on a high nutrient density diet. *Nutrition Journal.* 2010;9:51. doi:10.1186/1475-2891-9-51.

7. Camilleri GM, Méjean C, Bellisle F, Hercberg S, Péneau S. Association between Mindfulness and Weight Status in a General Population from the NutriNet-Santé Study. Gillison F, ed. *PLoS ONE.* 2015;10(6):e0127447. doi:10.1371/journal.pone.0127447.

8. Christaki E, Kokkinos A, Costarelli V, et al. Stress management can facilitate weight loss in Greek overweight and obese women: a pilot study. *J Hum Nutr Diet.* 2013; 26 (suppl 1):S132-139. doi: 101111/ jhn12086.

CHAPTER FIVE

PREVENTING AND REVERSING DIABETES

Diabetes is an all-too-personal time bomb which can go off today, tomorrow, next year, or ten years from now - a time bomb affecting millions like me and the children here today.

—MARY TYLER MOORE

I have high blood sugars, and Type 2 diabetes is not going to kill me. But I just have to eat right, and exercise, and lose weight, and watch what I eat, and I will be fine for the rest of my life.

—TOM HANKS

MR. JONES, FIFTY YEARS OLD, PRESENTED HIMSELF to my clinic with fatigue and increased abdominal girth. He was due for his annual exam. On follow-up blood work, his fasting blood sugar was 128 and his cholesterol was severely abnormal with triglycerides of 559. His waistline was 43 inches and his blood pressure was 149/93. He was surprised at his new diagnosis of diabetes and more surprised that his cholesterol was abnormal since he recently changed his diet. He told me he eats mostly fruits and veggies, and when I asked him how much fruits his reply was "Tons, Doc."

This patient was eating an excessive amount

of sugar from fruits. This led to increased weight gain and adiposity which led to insulin resistance, and the extra sugar in his diet was being converted to triglycerides. In this chapter, I will explore the nutritional principles that will help prevent and treat diabetes.

This case report about Mr. Jones represents a patient with metabolic syndrome. The American Heart Association defines the metabolic syndrome as abdominal obesity (waist circumference of 40 inches or above in men, and 35 inches or above in women), triglyceride level of 150 milligrams per deciliter of blood (mg/dL) or greater, HDL cholesterol of less than 40 mg/dL in men or less than 50 mg/dL in women, systolic blood pressure (top number) of 130 millimeters of mercury (mmHg) or greater, or diastolic blood pressure (bottom number) of 85 mm Hg or greater, fasting glucose of 100 mg/dL or greater. These risk factors, when clustered together, greatly increase the risk of heart disease and diabetes. In the above case, the patient has a fasting blood sugar of 128. This value is above the cut-off point for a diagnosis of diabetes. Let's explore the economic burden, causes, definition, and ways to treat and prevent diabetes.

The American Diabetic Association estimates that the total cost of treating diabetics in 2012 was an astonishing 245 billion dollars! According to the Center for Disease Control, by 2050, one out of three Americans may have diabetes. There are certain time-honored activities that are free, for example exercising and daily fasting, for maintaining an appropriate weight that can prevent and even reverse diabetes. Furthermore, if we heed Hippocrates's wisdom of letting food be our medicine, we can drastically reduce or avoid the economic burden that diabetes has placed on society. It is ironic that with all the sophisticated tools that we have to diagnose diabetes and the advanced methods of treating it, we are still quite ignorant as a society when it comes to focusing on the prevention of diabetes. Let us explore a brief history of this disease, one of the leading causes of death and afflicts millions of Americans.

First, what is diabetes mellitus? Diabetes mellitus is a condition of abnormal blood sugar metabolism. The word diabetes comes from the Greek root meaning "passing through." The word mellitus comes from the Latin root meaning "honey-sweet." So then, the term diabetes mellitus literally means "passing through" "honey-sweet" (urine). Indeed, in ancient times that is how physicians diagnosed diabetes, namely, by tasting the sweet urine of patients that were very sick. Although diabetes mellitus has been described for many thousands of years, as far back as Ancient Egypt in 1500 BC, its pathophysiology or cause remained a mystery for thousands of years. Before the discovery of insulin in the early 1920s by Canadian scientists Banting and Best, patients with diabetes lived very short lives and died very painful deaths. Type 1 diabetes usually presents in children and is due to a complete insulin deficiency. Whereas type 2 diabetes usually presents in adulthood and is strongly associated with adiposity and obesity. Over 2000 years ago, this observation was made by Ayurvedic physicians Sushruta and Charaka. The Ayurvedic text, *Charaka Samhita*, describes a method of diagnosing diabetes mellitus through mere observation alone. If the urine looked like honey and attracted ants and flies, then one could conclude that there was sugar in the urine and blood according to this astute clinical observation. These ancient physicians also emphasized that it is better to prevent this disease than to try to treat it. Indeed, this is salient advice not only for the health of the individual, but for the financial well-being of our country. To get a better understanding of how to prevent and treat diabetes, let's dive into and fully understand the pathophysiology of diabetes.

The underlying cause of type 1 diabetes is the result of autoimmune destruction of insulin-producing cells in the pancreas. The process is multifactorial and may involve genetic susceptibility, viral infections, and dietary factors such as cow's milk and cereals. Since we cannot control the genes one is born with and the childhood viruses one is exposed to, let's focus our attention on dietary factors. A study from Finland suggests that introducing dairy at a young age and high milk consumption during childhood increases the likelihood of developing type 1 diabetes.[1] The proposed mechanism is cow's protein promoting an immune response and antibody formation. These antibodies are formed to attack the invader, i.e. cow's protein. Since this protein has a similar molecular structure to the pancreas cells, these antibodies end up attacking and eventually destroying the pancreas. The end result is insulin dependent diabetes or type 1 diabetes. Vitamin D and omega-3 fatty acids can offer some protection against type 1 diabetes, and we shall explore this further in the treatment section.

The mechanism of type 2 diabetes is quite different and is directly related to obesity and insulin resistance. There is a new term known as diabesity, which literally is diabetes that comes on as a complication of obesity. This happens over long periods of time and over many insults to the pancreas. Type 2 diabetes is strongly influenced by genetics since we know that African Americans, Hispanics and Native Americans have a two to six times greater risk of diabetes than Caucasians in the U.S.[2] Furthermore, U.S. Pima Indians are five times more likely to have diabetes than Pima Indians in Mexico.[3] Also, twin studies show that if one twin has type 2 diabetes, than the other twin is 90 percent likely to develop diabetes in their lifetime. However, there is an abundance of evidence that shows with lifestyle alone, you can completely avoid this disease, even if you are genetically predisposed. Simple measures such as daily exercise, weight maintenance, and dietary modification can help you avoid the initial stages that lead to diabetes type 2, namely excessive adipose and insulin resistance.

Insulin resistance is, by definition, when insulin has less sensitivity (ability to import glucose into the cells for energy) which leads to increased secretion of insulin from the pancreas. Insulin resistance is an excellent predictor of type 2 diabetes and is closely linked to obesity. Adipose tissue (fat cells) are metabolically active and release hormones such as leptin, adiponectin, tumor necrosis factor alpha and resistin to name a few, that contribute to insulin resistance. In sum, there is a vicious cycle: A poor diet with high amounts of sugar increases adipose tissue, which leads to increased blood sugar, which increases insulin secretion, which leads to decreased insulin sensitivity (resistance), which over time leads to type 2 diabetes.

A person with diabetes usually feels normal or asymptomatic. This may surprise many readers. Since greater than 90 percent of diabetics have type 2, which is associated with insulin resistance and excessive adipose (fat) in the initial stages of their disease, they will be asymptomatic. Indeed, most type 2 diabetics have had their disease for ten years before a doctor diagnoses them. In contrast, most type 1 diabetics present extremely sick and are in a life-threatening condition unless treated with insulin and IV fluids. Both types 1 and 2 can present with the classic symptoms of hypergly-cemia (elevated blood sugar). These symptoms include excessive urination (polyuria), excessive thirst (polydipsia), excessive hunger (polyphagia), blurred vision and weight loss to name a few. Some patients present in a life threatening coma from diabetic ketoacidosis and need care in an intensive care unit. These patients are said to be, "starving in the sea of plenty." This is because they can have extremely elevated blood sugar, which is a form of potential energy for the body (sea of plenty), yet they are starving because they have no insulin to bring this energy into the cells. Some may present to their doctor's office with vague symptoms of fatigue and not feeling well. It is the relative state of insu-lin in the body that will determine how dramatic or life threatening the presentation is. In sum, the clinical presentation of a diabetic patient depends on the amount of functional insulin present. In the severe life threatening cases, there is no functional insulin. In other cases, the degree of presentation will be directly proportional to the degree of insulin resistance.

How does someone get officially diagnosed with diabetes? There are several ways to diagnose. One scenario is if someone has the classic symptoms of hyperglycemia (mentioned previously) and a random blood sugar of 200 or higher. Another method is a fasting morning blood sugar of greater than 126. Also, an oral glucose challenge where a patient drinks a 75 gram solution of sugar water and if the blood sugar is equal to or greater than 200. Finally, a blood test known as a hemoglobin A1C of equal to or greater than 6.5. Any abnormal lab test should be repeated to confirm the diagnosis.

Let us explore the natural and holistic treatment of diabetes without the use of pharmaceuticals. The best diet to treat, reverse, and prevent diabetes is a whole foods, low glycemic, plant-based diet. In other words, based on the best available science, a vegan diet is the best diet to prevent and reverse diabetes. Ideally, at least 50 to 66 percent raw and organic and 100 percent from plants. It should be raw to preserve more of the phytonutrients and enzymes that can be denatured through high heat cooking. It should be organic to avoid pesticides that have been linked to neurologic disease such as Parkinson's Disease.[4] Again, the diet should be vegan and avoid all animal products, including eggs. A recent study published in May 2013 shows that daily egg consumption increased the risk of diabetes.[5] It was a prospective study of about 20,000 men and 36,000 women, and the data suggests an association between daily egg consumption and type 2 diabetes in men and women. Many people are aware of the association between red meat consumption and cancer, heart disease and strokes, but are unaware of the data linking red meat consumption and diabetes. A study published in 2010 in the journal *Circulation* shows that the biggest culprit is processed meats and its link to heart disease and diabetes. It's no wonder that as Americans' love affair with processed meats such as salami, pepperoni, ham, and hot dogs has increased, the incidence of diabetes has skyrocketed to 29.1 million Americans, or 9.3 percent of the population.[6] It's not just processed meats, but plain red meat intake from hamburgers and steaks is also associated with increased risk of diabetes type 2.[7] The pathophysiology may involve the fact that meat causes a very high insulin spike comparable to processed sugar. Moreover, research from Harvard School of Public Health postulates that sodium, nitrites, and iron are also culprits in the pathophysiology of diabetes type 2. Further, dairy consumption should be avoided, since it has long been linked to type 1 diabetes.[8] Ironically, the ADA (American Diabetic Association) diet is inferior to other diets, and the amount of carbohydrates consumed may hold the clues as to why.

Evidence suggests that relative carbohydrate restriction is effective in treating diabetes and helping with weight loss.[9] A low carbohydrate diet is defined as consuming less than 130 grams of carbohydrates per day or 26 percent energy from carbohydrates. However, ADA recommends approximately 185 to 230 grams of carbohydrates per day or approximately 45 percent energy from carbohydrates. By eating a whole foods plant-based diet, one can effortlessly achieve a moderate-carbohydrate diet: 26–45 percent. A recent study showed that a vegan low-carbohydrate 'Eco-Atkins' diet of about 130 grams of carbs per day was more effective than a standard high-carbohydrate lacto-ovo vegetarian diet in improving lipids.[10]

The foods that should be consumed should be from 100 percent plant origin since they are naturally low glycemic and relatively lower in carbohydrates. As previously noted, animal foods are associated with increased risk of diabetes, but we now know that plant foods such as fruits and vegetables help prevent diabetes.[11]

Another great food to consume regularly is beans. Beans have been shown to not only lower cholesterol and blood pressure, but they provide an excellent way to lower blood sugar.[12] Furthermore, not only do beans help blood sugar metabolism, they help to control satiety and help decrease inflammation.[13]

The ADA diet has been compared to a vegan diet in a head-to-head comparison to see which diet was better at controlling blood sugar. In this study published in the American Journal of Clinical Nutrition, a low-fat vegan diet was superior to the standard ADA diet. A review of the literature shows that a vegan diet is more effective treatment for type 2 diabetes than the conventional medical paradigm of pharmaceuticals.[14]

In the *Adventist Health Study 2* published in 2013 there was a direct correlation between meat consumption and diabetes.[15] This study involved almost 90,000 subjects, and any meat consumption increased the risk of developing diabetes. Vegans had the lowest risk. Furthermore, Dr. Neal Barnard, M.D., and colleagues published a recent study comparing a low-fat vegan diet to a conventional ADA diet in the treatment of type 2 diabetes. The low-fat vegan diet was more effective at controlling blood sugar and plasma lipids.[16]

In short, a plant-based diet rich in antioxidants, B vitamins, minerals, and phytonutrients and that is 100 percent plant-based or vegan is the best way to treat or reverse diabetes. A vegan diet provides all the phytonutrients and minerals and vitamins necessary to maintain an optimal weight and regulate blood sugar metabolism. A plant-based diet rich in antioxidants, B vitamins, complex carbohydrates, minerals, and phytonutrients is the best way to treat or reverse diabetes type 2. This diet provides the phytonutrients and minerals and vitamins necessary to maintain an optimal weight, regulate blood sugar metabolism, prevent and even reverse diabetes mellitus type 2! What is the best diet to maintain an optimal weight? Let's explore this further.

According to the CDC, 35.7 percent of the U.S. population is obese. As previously discussed, a huge risk factor for developing diabetes type 2 is obesity and insulin resistance, which leads to diabetes. One of the most important dietary interventions one can make to lose weight is avoiding meat. All meats including red meat, chicken, and processed meats are associated with weight gain.[17]

Vegans have the lowest BMI or healthy lean weight and the lowest risk of developing type 2 diabetes. In a study from the Seventh Day Adventists, more than 60,000 subjects were analyzed. There were meat eaters, semi-vegetarians, pesco-vegetarians, lacto-ovo vegetarians, and vegans. All diet types in this study were in the overweight BMI, and only the vegans maintained a healthy lean BMI of less than 25.[18] Chicken consumption is associated with increased weight gain and a higher BMI.[19] A prospective study that followed a total of 103,455 men and 270,348 women aged twenty-five to seventy from ten European countries showed the following: Total meat (red meat, chicken, and processed meat) intakes were all "positively associated with weight gain after an average of five years of follow-up." What is amazing is that the results were statistically significant after adjusting for calorie intake, physical activity, and dietary pattern.

If the risk of developing diabetes from being overweight or obese is not enough of an incentive to get healthy, here is another reason. According to The National Cancer Institute, increasing BMI and fat cells increases one's risk of cancer by increasing estrogen, insulin, IGF-1, adipokines, oxidative stress, and inflammation. The cancers associated with obesity are: esophagus, pancreas, colon and rectum, breast (after menopause), endometrium (lining of the uterus), kidney, thyroid, gallbladder, and possibly others.[20]

A vegan diet that allows for optimal weight maintenance and provides adequate phytonutrients, vitamins, healthy fats, and minerals will enhance and promote healthy glucose metabolism. Therefore, based on the best available evidence, a vegan diet is the best method to prevent, treat, and reverse diabetes. There are several "styles" of vegan diets that I will summarize below.

Several physicians have had great results with reversing diabetes through diet alone. Gabriel Cousens, M.D., has a 30-day program at the Tree of Life in Arizona with an excellent success rate. In his movie, *Simply Raw, Reversing Diabetes in 30 days*, he uses a 100 percent raw food vegan diet and is able to cure diabetes even in patients who are on insulin. He has data on 120 patients that shows a 61 percent cure rate (no insulin) on type 2 diabetes and a 21 percent cure rate of type 1 diabetes. This approach is a diet that is 100 percent raw food or live food with no consumption of animal products. The seeds, nuts, beans, and grains are sprouted to help activate enzymes and multiplies its nutritional profile up to fifteen times its original content. The fruits and greens on this program are organic and eaten fresh and raw. Recipes available for this diet include pizza, hummus, breads, pasta, burgers, cakes, and pies! All of these recipes involve only plants in their natural states.

Joel Fuhrman, M.D., is also a nutrition expert

who uses a diet that is high nutrient and low calorie known as a nutritarian diet. The approach allows for up to 10 percent of the diet to come from animal sources, but he encourages a 100 percent plant source for optimal results. I also encourage my patients to avoid animal foods since they offer very little nutritional benefits. Furthermore, there is a strong association between red meat consumption and increased risk of diabetes as shown in a Harvard study.[21] Also, meat consumption is associated with weight gain. Weight gain and increase in adipose tissue (fat cells) is one of the main mechanisms of insulin resistance and type 2 diabetes. This nutritarian diet, or 100 percent vegan diet is, by definition, low calorie and low glycemic, but extremely high in phytonutrients.

Some unique features of Dr. Fuhrman's approach is that he strongly encourages an avoidance of refined oils and any added salts. It is known that humans generate completely new taste buds in just three weeks. So, after a change in diet, in just three weeks, the foods in their natural unadulterated state will taste salty or sweet or bitter, etc. Also, beans are a fantastic source of vegan protein. Beans, according to a recent study, lower one's blood sugar and decrease insulin secretion and visceral fat.[22] One of the reasons beans are extremely healthy is because the carbohydrates in beans are a resistant starch and functions as a fiber. One of my favorite books for reversing and preventing diabetes is *The*

End Of Diabetes by Dr. Joel Fuhrman, M.D.

There are some supplements that could be used as adjuncts to a whole-food, plant-based diet that help with blood sugar metabolism. Research shows there is a statistically significant improvement in blood sugar and cholesterol with the consumption of cinnamon.[23] I recommend ceylon cinnamon since it is safe and effective, and one level teaspoon is adequate for its health promoting benefits. One should avoid cassia cinnamon since it may contain high levels of a toxin coumarin that could cause liver damage. Ceylon cinnamon also has anti-inflammatory and antibacterial properties.

Chromium is an essential mineral that is crucial for blood sugar metabolism, and up to 50 percent of the population is deficient. This important nutrient helps prevent insulin resistance and actually improves insulin sensitivity.[24] Through the food processing industry, this essential trace mineral is stripped from foods. Chromium's bioavailability is increased with vitamin C but even still, less than 2 percent of chromium is absorbed. It is found naturally occurring in foods such as onions, tomatoes, potatoes, lettuce, broccoli, grapes, and whole grains. A whole-food, plant-based diet provides adequate chromium from foods, but diabetics should consider taking this supplement. Chromium is also important in developing lean muscles and reducing adipose tissue. Athletes are at higher risk of deficiency. I recommend up to 200 mcg of chromium per day for diabetics and athletes in consultation with your physician. For insulin dependent diabetics, glucose blood levels should be monitored more closely since chromium increases insulin sensitivity and blood sugar may drop.

Another mineral that is important in glucose metabolism is magnesium. Magnesium is involved in over 300 chemical reactions in the body and important for nerve, bone, and muscle function. There is a significant association between higher intakes of magnesium and a reduced risk of diabetes.[25] I recommend getting magnesium from foods such as green leafy vegetables, legumes, nuts, soybeans, avocados, and brown rice. Diabetics should consider taking 400 mg daily of magnesium glycinate with food, in consultation with a physician to help monitor blood sugars.

Zinc is a mineral that has shown promising effects in lower blood sugar and is a powerful antioxidant. Zinc is a cofactor for more than 300 enzymes and is needed for cell growth, reproduction, immune function, vision, wound healing, and collagen. A systematic review and meta-analysis on the effects of zinc supplementation in patients with diabetes showed a beneficial effects on blood sugar control and lipids.[26] Daily dosage of zinc is 15 to 30 mg per day depending on your diet, in consultation with a physician. Healthy sources of zinc include legumes, chocolate, nuts, pumpkin seeds, and whole grains.

Coenzyme Q10 (CoQ10) is a ubiquitous antioxidant found in every cell in the human body. It is necessary for energy production in the mitochondria. This compound helps reduce oxidative stress, improved endothelial function, decrease fatigue, improves blood flow, and lowers blood sugar and blood pressure.[27] Any patient with a history of chronic fatigue syndrome, metabolic syndrome, hypertension, heart disease, on a statin, and wanting to decrease oxidation should consider taking this supplement. The healthiest sources of CoQ10 are peanuts, sesame seeds, pistachios, broccoli, cauliflower, oranges, strawberries, and legumes. I recommend taking 120 mg of CoQ10 once daily with food.

Another exciting supplement that should be considered by all diabetics and prediabetics is berberine. Berberine is comparable to oral diabetic pharmaceuticals in controlling blood sugar and dyslipidemia.[28,29] Berberine (Oregon Grape) is an herbal compound with anti-inflammatory and anti-diabetic properties. Berberine should be taken 500 mg with meals three times a day with consultation with your doctor in diabetic patients.

Also, alpha lipoic acid is a powerful antioxidant found naturally in spinach and broccoli that helps with blood sugar metabolism. It is essential for energy production and helps fight free radicals. There is strong evidence it helps to treat the symptoms of diabetic neuropathy. There are studies showing it decreases general oxidation and blood sugar.[30,31] I recommend alpha lipoic acid in a dose of 300mg daily in consultation with a physician for diabetics.

Amla, or Indian gooseberry, is a fruit from India that has one of the highest antioxidant contents of any food. Amla plays a central role in Ayurvedic medicine and is found in the popular remedy triphala. In a recent study, it was shown to lower blood sugar better than glyburide, a modern pharmaceutical used to treat type 2 diabetes.[32] In diabetic patients, just three teaspoons of dried amla powder was more effective than glyburide in lowering blood sugar.

All patients, especially those with diabetes should ensure adequate vitamin D supplementation since a recent study showed a link between low vitamin D levels and all cause mortality in patients with type 1 diabetes.[33] Furthermore, not only should adults get adequate vitamin D to optimize blood sugar metabolism, but infants and children should supplement with vitamin D to help prevent type 1 diabetes.[34] Breast-fed infants should supplement with 400 I.U. of vitamin D since breast milk does not provide enough unless the mother is supplementing in large doses. I recommend daily vitamin D of 1000 I.U. to 3000 I.U. depending on sun exposure, season, geographical location, age, and current blood levels.

One compound that is often overlooked but has a powerful effect on blood sugar is dietary fiber. The American diet is woefully inadequate in dietary fiber. We have known for decades that increasing dietary fiber in one's diet has beneficial effects on lipids and blood sugar. A randomized trial published in the *New England Journal of Medicine* compared the standard ADA diet (24 grams of fiber) with a high fiber diet (50 grams of daily fiber.) The results were impressive for the high-fiber diet. The high-fiber diet group had a 24-hour plasma glucose lowered by 10 percent and cholesterol, triglycerides, and LDL cholesterol lowered by as much as 12.5 percent.[35] If one follows a whole-food, plant-based diet, obtaining 50 g daily dietary fiber comes with relative ease.

In summary, we have conclusive evidence of the dietary factors that can prevent and treat diabetes. Plant foods help one maintain an optimal body weight and avoid obesity, which is a major risk factor for developing diabetes. However, even in those who maintain a normal body weight, meat consumption has been associated with increasing the risk of diabetes, and plant consumption decreases risk. There are also several safe and effective supplements that should be considered by all diabetics in consultation with a physician.

PEARLS FROM CHAPTER 5

By 2050, one out of three Americans will have diabetes and it costs billions of dollars to treat. The great news is there is an effective modality to treat and prevent diabetes that is free of any side effects.

The best method to reverse and prevent diabetes is an organic whole foods, low-glycemic, plant-based-diet. The diet should be rich in cooked and raw vegetables, legumes, nuts, seeds, and fruits. For optimal health avoid refined grains, oils, and animal products. Also, diabetics should consider taking certain supplements such as cinnamon, chromium, magnesium, CoQ10, Alpha Lipoic Acid, and berberine that have shown beneficial results in blood sugar metabolism in consultation with a physician.

Chapter 5 endnotes

1. Virtanen SM, Saukkonen T, Savilahti E, et al. Diet, cow's milk protein antibodies and the risk of IDDM in Finnish children Childhood Diabetes in Finland Study Group. *Diabetologia*.1994;37(4):381-387.

2. Caprio S, Daniels SR, Drewnowski A, et al. Influence of Race, Ethnicity, and Culture on Childhood Obesity: Implications for Prevention and Treatment: A consensus statement of Shaping America's Health and the Obesity Society. *Diabetes Care*. 2008;31(11):2211-2221. doi:10.2337/dc08-9024.

3. Baier LJ, Hanson RL. Genetic studies of the etiology of type 2 diabetes in Pima Indians: hunting for pieces to a complicated puzzle. *Diabetes*. 2004;53(5):1181-1186.

4. Wang A, Costello S, Cockburn M, Zhang X, Bronstein J, Ritz B. Parkinson's disease risk from ambient exposure to pesticides. *European journal of epidemiology*. 2011;26(7):547-555. doi:10.1007/s10654-011-9574-5.

5. Shin JY, Xun P, Nakamura Y, He K. Egg consumption in

relation to risk of cardiovascular disease and diabetes: a systematic review and meta-analysis. *The American Journal of Clinical Nutrition.* 2013;98(1):146-159. doi:10.3945/ajcn.112.051318.

6. 2014 National Diabetes Statistics Report. Centers for Disease Control and Prevention website. http://www.cdc.gov/diabetes/data/statistics/2014statisticsreport.html.

7. Bendinelli B, Palli D, Masala G, et al. Association between dietary meat consumption and incident type 2 diabetes: the EPIC-InterAct study.InterAct Consortium. *Diabetologia.* 2013; 56(1):47-59. doi: 101007/s00125-012-2718-7.

8. Gottlieb, S. Early Exposure to cows' milk raises risk of diabetes in high risk children. *BMJ.* 2000;321:1040. doi: 10.1136/bmj.321.7268.1040/d.

9. Feinman RD, Pogozelski WK, Astrup A, et al. Dietary carbohydrate restriction as the first approach in diabetes management: critical review and evidence base. *Nutrition.* 2015;31(1):1-13. doi: 101016/jnut201406011.

10. Jenkins DJA, Wong JMW, Kendall CWC, et al. Effect of a 6-month vegan low-carbohydrate ("Eco-Atkins") diet on cardiovascular risk factors and body weight in hyperlipidaemic adults: a randomised controlled trial. *BMJ Open.* 2014;4(2):e003505. doi:10.1136/bmjopen-2013-003505.

11. Cooper AJ, Sharp SJ, Lentjes MA, et al. A prospective study of the association between quantity and variety of fruit and vegetable intake and incident type 2 diabetes. *Diabetes Care.* 2012;35(6):1293-1300. doi:10.2337/dc11-2388.

12. Jenkins DA, Kendall CC, Augustin LA, et al. Effect of Legumes as Part of a Low Glycemic Index Diet on Glycemic Control and Cardiovascular Risk Factors in Type 2

Diabetes Mellitus: A Randomized Controlled Trial. *Arch Intern Med.* 2012;172(21):1653-1660. doi:10.1001/2013. jamainternmed.70.

13. Nilsson A, Johansson E, Ekström L, Björck I. Effects of a Brown Beans Evening Meal on Metabolic Risk Markers and Appetite Regulating Hormones at a Subsequent Standardized Breakfast: A Randomized Cross-Over Study. Blachier F, ed. *PLoS ONE.* 2013;8(4):e59985. doi:10.1371/ journal.pone.0059985.

14. Barnard ND, Katcher HI, Jenkins DJ, Cohen J, Turner-McGrievy G. Vegetarian and vegan diets in type 2 diabetes management. *Nutr Rev.* 2009;67(5):255-263. doi: 101111/ j1753- 4887200900198x.

15. Orlich MJ, Singh P, Sabaté J, et al. Vegetarian Dietary Patterns and Mortality in Adventist Health Study 2. *JAMA Intern Med.* 2013;173(13):1230-1238. doi:10.1001/jamainternmed.2013.6473.

16. Barnard ND, Cohen J, Jenkins DJ, et al. A low-fat vegan diet and a conventional diabetes diet in the treatment of type 2 diabetes: a randomized, controlled, 74-wk clinical trial. *The American Journal of Clinical Nutrition.* 2009;89(5):1588S-1596S. doi:10.3945/ajcn.2009.26736H.

17. Vergnaud AC, Norat T, Romaguera D, et al. Meat consumption and prospective weight change in participants of the EPIC-PANACEA study. *Am J Clin Nutr.* 2010;92(2):398-407. doi: 103945/ ajcn200928713.

18. Tonstad S, Butler T, Yan R, Fraser GE. Type of Vegetarian Diet, Body Weight, and Prevalence of Type 2 Diabetes. *Diabetes Care.* 2009;32(5):791-796. doi:10.2337/dc08-1886.

19. Gilsing AM, Weijenberg MP, Hughes LA, et al. Longitu-

dinal Changes in BMI in Older Adults Are Associated with Meat Consumption Differentially, by Type of Meat Consumed. *J. Nutr.* 2012; 142(2): 340-349.

20. Obesity and Cancer Risk. NIH National Cancer Institute website. http://www.cancer.gov/cancertopics/factsheet/Risk/obesity.

21. Pan A, Sun Q, Bernstein AM, Manson JE, Willett WC, Hu FB. Changes in Red Meat Consumption and Subsequent Risk of Type 2 Diabetes: Three Cohorts of US Men and Women. *JAMA internal medicine.* 2013;173(14):1328-1335. doi:10.1001/jamainternmed.2013.6633.

22. Ventura E, Davis J, Byrd-Williams C, et al. Reduction in Risk Factors for Type 2 Diabetes Mellitus in Response to a Low-Sugar, High-Fiber Dietary Intervention in Overweight Latino Adolescents. *Archives of pediatrics & adolescent medicine.* 2009;163(4):320-327. doi:10.1001/archpediatrics.2009.11.

23. Allen RW, Schwartzman E, Baker WL, Coleman CI, Phung OJ. Cinnamon Use in Type 2 Diabetes: An Updated Systematic Review and Meta-Analysis. *Annals of Family Medicine.* 2013;11(5):452-459. doi:10.1370/afm.1517.

24. Wang ZQ, Cefalu WT. Current concepts about chromium supplementation in type 2 diabetes and insulin resistance. *Curr Diab.* 2010;10(2):145-151. doi: 101007/ s11892-010-0097-3.

25. Dong J-Y, Xun P, He K, Qin L-Q. Magnesium Intake and Risk of Type 2 Diabetes: Meta-analysis of prospective cohort studies. *Diabetes Care.* 2011;34(9):2116-2122. doi:10.2337/dc11-0518.

26. Jayawardena R, Ranasinghe P, Galappatthy P, Malkanthi R,

Constantine G, Katulanda P. Effects of zinc supplementation on diabetes mellitus: a systematic review and meta-analysis. *Diabetology & Metabolic Syndrome*. 2012;4:13. doi:10.1186/1758-5996-4-13.

27. Hodgson JM, Watts GF, Playford DA, Burke V, Croft KD. Coenzyme Q10 improves blood pressure and glycaemic control: a controlled trial in subjects with type 2 diabetes. *Eur J Clin Nutr*. 2002;56(11):1137-1142.

28. Dong H, Wang N, Zhao L, Lu F. Berberine in the Treatment of Type 2 Diabetes Mellitus: A Systemic Review and Meta-Analysis. *Evidence-based Complementary and Alternative Medicine* : eCAM. 2012;2012:591654. doi:10.1155/2012/591654.

29. Yin J, Xing H, Ye J. Efficacy of Berberine in Patients with Type 2 Diabetes. Metabolism: clinical and experimental. 2008;57(5):712-717. doi:10.1016/j.metabol.2008.01.013.

30. Golbidi S, Badran M, Laher I. Diabetes and Alpha Lipoic Acid. *Frontiers in Pharmacology*. 2011;2:69. doi:10.3389/fphar.2011.00069.

31. Gomes MB, Negrato CA. Alpha-lipoic acid as a pleiotropic compound with potential therapeutic use in diabetes and other chronic diseases. *Diabetology & Metabolic Syndrome*. 2014;6:80. doi:10.1186/1758-5996-6-80.

32. D'souza JJ, D'souza PP, Fazal F, Kumar A, Bhat HP, Baliga MS. Anti-diabetic effects of the Indian indigenous fruit Emblica officinalis Gaertn: active constituents and modes of action. *Food Funct*. 2014;5(4):635-644. doi: 10.1039/c3fo60366k.

33. Mathieu C, Bart J Van der Schueren. Vitamin D Deficiency Is Not Good for You. *Diabetes Care*. 2011;34(5):1245-1246.

34. Hyppönen E, Läärä E, Reunanen A, Järvelin MR, Virtanen SM. Intake of vitamin D and risk of type 1 diabetes: a birth-cohort study. *Lancet.* 2001;358(9292):1500-1503.

35. Chandalia M, Garg A, Lutjohann D, von Bergmann K, Grundy SM, Brinkley LJ. Beneficial effects of high dietary fiber intake in patients with type 2 diabetes mellitus. *N Engl J Med.* 2000;342(19):1392-1398.

CHAPTER SIX

Preventing and Reversing Heart Disease

Think about it: Heart disease and diabetes, which account for more deaths in the U.S. and worldwide than everything else combined, are completely preventable by making comprehensive lifestyle changes. Without drugs or surgery.

—Dean Ornish, M.D.

I saw many people who had advanced heart disease and I was so frustrated because I knew if they just knew how to do the right thing, simple lifestyle and diet steps, that the entire trajectory of their life and health would have been different.

—Mehmet Oz, M.D.

Ms. Randall is a forty-nine-year-old female, avid runner who suffered a major myocardial infarction (heart attack). She required a stent to help save her life. She came to me and asked me if a plant-based diet would help reverse her heart disease. I said, "Yes." After thirty months on a plant-based diet, her coronary angiogram showed reversal of her coronary artery disease (CAD).

CAD is atherosclerosis that affects the coronary arteries that supply oxygen and nutrients to myocardial tissue. When the coronary artery gets clogged, it leads to a myocardial infarction (MI) or a heart attack. CAD is known as a silent killer because many times patients are asymptomatic. The first "symptom" of chest pain can lead to sudden cardiac death from an MI. Some are lucky enough to experience warning symptoms such as chest pain with exertion, also known as angina.

The pathophysiology of CAD is complex and there is no unifying hypothesis in the medical community. We know the modifiable risk factors that contribute to CAD worldwide in both sexes include hypertension, diabetes, dyslipidemia, smoking, abdominal obesity, psychosocial factors, underconsumption of fruits and vegetables, overconsumption of alcohol, and lack of regular physical activity.[1] Also, endothelial dysfunction, inflammation, immunologic factors, and plaque rupture play a role. Most prepubescent children, by the age of ten years old, have numerous macrophage foam cells and fatty streaks seen on inner lining of the coronary arteries. It is astonishing to note that in America, a child by the age of ten years old has CAD with fatty streaks visible on the coronary arteries.[2] It is a sad fact that heart disease is so epidemic in America that we have risk calculators that help determine the likelihood of an advanced atherosclerotic lesion in pediatric patients.[3] Although heart disease has been the leading cause of death in America for almost 100 years, many experts and epidemiological studies support the claim that coronary heart disease is preventable. Also, we know that through intensive lifestyle intervention, heart disease is reversible.[4,5]

Cardiovascular disease is a worldwide epidemic. It has been the leading cause of death in America since 1912, and in the top three causes of death since 1901. In most developed countries, cardiovascular disease is the number one killer. The prevalence of heart disease is also increasing in developing countries.[6] We have known for years that heart disease starts at a very early age as conclusively shown by the Korean Soldier Study.[7] In this landmark study, 300 American soldiers who died in the Korean war were autopsied. The average age was twenty-two and an astounding 77.3 percent of hearts showed evidence of atherosclerosis. The Korean men's hearts were examined, and the investigators noted a lack of blockages and attributed it to dietary factors.

The CDC reports that 26.6 million people in the United States have CAD. That number does not include the millions of children and young adults in the undetected early stages of heart disease. We know that heart disease is the leading cause of death in both men and women and kills about 600,000 people annually in the U.S. or about one in every four deaths.[8] Every year about 715,000 Americans have a heart attack, and the US spends 108.9 billion annually on healthcare expenditures for this preventable disease.[9]

Our knowledge over the past sixty years has advanced tremendously, and today we can clearly identify risk factors for cardiovascular disease. Some of the classic risk factors include cigarette smoking, diabetes, dyslipidemia, hypertension, male age greater than forty-five and female age greater than fifty-five, and family history of premature heart disease. Other risk factors include obesity, hyperglycemia, sedentary lifestyle, red meat consumption, high fat dairy, high glycemic diet, psychiatric disorder, and chronic stress.

There are several ways to diagnosis heart disease. The following biochemical markers can be indicative of heart disease: Troponin I and CPK-MB are serum markers of myocardial infarction (heart attack). Brain natriuretic peptide (BNP) can be a sign of congestive heart failure (CHF). The lipid profile including total cholesterol, LDL (low-density lipoprotein), or "bad" cholesterol, HDL (high-density lipoprotein), or "good" cholesterol, and triglycerides. Also, C-reactive protein (CRP) and homocysteine are markers of inflammation and increased cardiac risk.

Non-invasive measure include a simple chest X-ray for clues of cardiomegaly (enlarged heart). Electrocardiogram (EKG) shows the electrical activity of the heart. An echocardiogram is an ultrasound of the heart, measuring heart function. Stress ECG, echocardiography, or the nuclear stress test are advanced cardiac tests that determine how the heart performs under stress. These non-invasive tests can help evaluate heart function, valves, heart size, electrical conduction, and evidence of new or old heart injury. There is a newer imaging modality called the cardiac computed tomography that gives a coronary calcium scoring. This calcium score helps predict the risk of heart disease.

The gold standard still remains an invasive test called the cardiac catheterization and coronary angiography. This procedure gives a direct visualization of the coronary arteries and helps determine if the blood vessels have narrowed or are blocked. Finally, it is a sad fact that many people are diagnosed with coronary artery disease on autopsy, as it is a stealthy silent killer.

Standard treatment in contemporary cardiology is usually pharmaceutical drugs to control blood pressure, diabetes, and lipids. Using pharmaceutical interventions is not without side effects. Let's take Lipitor, which has generated billions of dollars in profit for the pharmaceutical industry, and is used to lower cholesterol. Some serious side effects from taking Lipitor include rhabdomyolysis, acute renal failure, hepatotoxicity, pancreatitis, life threatening skin rash, diabetes, and cognitive impairment. If coronary artery disease advances, then invasive procedures such as angioplasty and coronary artery bypass graft are employed. As the esteemed Professor of Cardiology, Dr. Caldwell Esselstyn, M.D. so aptly points out, modern medicine is more concerned with treating symptoms than finding and curing the underlying disease. In his fascinating article, Dr. Esselstyn astutely calls the current treatment paradigm "palliative cardiology."[10] However, we have a current scientific approach that has been shown to prevent and reverse heart disease. The great thing about this approach is that it involves safe lifestyle interventions devoid of side effects.

We have a preponderance of data that suggests that eating fruits and vegetables prevents or decreases the risk of heart disease.[11-13] We also have a plethora of data that shows that a low-fat vegetarian diet can reverse heart disease.[4,14-17] No other diet in the history of mankind has been scientifically proven to reverse heart disease. From the science, we know that we can prevent heart disease and we can also reverse it once it is established. One prevalent, but flawed, argument is that heart disease is an inevitable part of the aging process. In many cultures, heart disease was rare until they adopted the unhealthy Western diet. In the Kitava Study, the Okinawa Study, the Seventh-day Adventist Health Study and the China Study, it was shown that populations that eat a predominantly plant-based diet and do not consume the highly processed Western diet have very low incidences of heart disease. In fact, some actually have no heart disease at a very advanced age!

Let us briefly explore this notion of a human being with no heart disease as we age. The reader may fancy this notion of no heart disease in an elder as a myth. We have data that shows one can grow to a ripe old age without heart disease. One of the last indigenous cultures in the world to live a lifestyle and have a strictly native diet not influenced by Western culture is the Kitava people. These indigenous people who live in Papua New Guinea only eat yams, sweet potatoes, taro, tapioca, bananas, papayas, pineapples, mangos, guava, watermelons, pumpkins, vegetables, fish, and coconuts.[18,19] In a study of 1,816 patients between the ages of three to ninety-six, it was noted that there was no ischemic heart disease.[20] This data was gathered by interviews, ECGs, and physical exams of living people, and it was reasonable to conclude that there was no heart disease.

Also, another landmark study on indigenous people from Uganda showed that heart disease was practically non-existent based on autopsy studies.[22] Even when the subjects were age matched with Missourians, the rate of heart disease was non-existent in Ugandans and was astonishingly high in Americans. An autopsy of the 632 Ugandans found only one myocardial infarction, and out of 632 Missourians, there were 136 myocardial infarction. The study controlled for confounding variables such as age and gender. In fact, out of 1,427 autopsies performed in this Ugandan study on subjects greater than forty years of age, only one small healed infarct was found.[21] In America, a sample of 1,427 autopsies will find heart disease as the cause of death in close to 500 cases! These findings are quite astonishing. What was the Ugandan secret to no heart disease?

Perhaps it was their diet? Indeed, it should be noted that the diet consumed by the Ugandans in this study was a whole-food, plant-based diet. The staple foods include green plantains, sweet potatoes, cassava, yams, maize, millet, pumpkins, beans, tomatoes, and green leafy vegetables.[22] It is reassuring to see these studies with elderly humans that are not afflicted with heart disease.

Furthermore, there is also an autopsy study of an Okinawan elder who was 100 years old, and her coronary arteries did not show any evidence of atherosclerosis.[23] Let me repeat that: No heart disease in a 100-year-old! This finding is so remarkable that I shall quote that portion of the article: "No atrial or ventricular dilatation or enlargement; no areas of infarction; no coronary artery calcification or atherosclerosis; no valvular calcification." As an aside, the study goes on to mention that the kidneys, esophagus, stomach, liver, pancreas, gallbladder, and bladder were essentially normal in this centenarian.

Although heart disease has been the leading cause of death in America for almost 100 years, many experts and epidemiological studies support the claim that coronary heart disease is preventable. Also, we know that through intensive lifestyle intervention, heart disease is reversible![15-17] As mentioned previously, heart disease is the leading cause of death in both men and women in America. Sadly, every year almost 1 million Americans have a heart attack and it is preventable by eating plants. In February 2015, the Dietary Guidelines Advisory Committee took a step in the right direction by recommending higher consumption of vegetables, fruits, whole grains, and a lower consumption of red and processed meat, and lower intakes of refined grains, and sugar-sweetened foods and beverages. Here is a direct quote from the Dietary Guidelines Advisory Committee: "The major findings regarding sustainable diets were that a diet higher in plant-based foods, such as vegetables, fruits, whole grains, legumes, nuts, and seeds, and lower in calories and animal-based foods is more health promoting. Current evidence shows that the average U.S. diet has a potentially larger environmental impact in terms of increased GHG emissions, land use, water use, and energy use, compared to the above dietary patterns."

The first line of defense against preventing coronary heart disease is a whole-food, plant-based diet. However, I would like to mention a supplement that should be considered in certain situations in consultation with your physician. A recent meta-analysis of twenty-seven original studies found an association between higher alpha-linolenic acid (short chain omega-3 fatty acid) and moderately lower risk of cardiovascular disease.[24] We know that C-reactive protein (CRP), is a marker of systemic inflammation and is linked to heart disease. A diet rich in alpha-linolenic acid can help decrease inflammation and decrease the risk of cardiovascular disease.[25]

I recommend taking 1-2 tablespoons of organic ground flax seeds daily and avoid refined oils.

Long chain fatty acids DHA/EPA, such the ones found in fish and algae offer numerous health benefits. Dietary short chain fatty acids, alpha-linolenic acid (ALA), can be converted to DHA/EPA but conversion is limited to 0 to 8 percent. Thus, it is important to consume DHA/EPA regularly and not rely on endogenous conversion. DHA/EPA can help decrease triglycerides, decrease blood pressure, decrease endothelial dysfunction, decrease thrombosis, and increase myocardial efficiency.[26] In short, regular consumption of DHA/EPA in one's diet can help with cardiovascular health by preventing progression of atherosclerosis, decreasing the risks of coronary restenosis, myocardial infarction, and sudden cardiac death.[27-29] Furthermore, DHA/EPA is important for eye health and may help prevent the leading cause of blindness in America, macular degeneration. Also, it is important for brain health. I have concerns about regular consumption of fish because of the potential risk of methylmercury, dioxins, polychlorinated biphenyls, polybrominated diphenyl ethers, and pesticides. Although commercially available fish oils remove these pollutants, I do not recommend fish oil because of the long-term sustainability and the negative environmental impact. I recommend 250 mg of micro-algae derived DHA/EPA daily.

There is sufficient evidence to prove that humans

can live a long and healthy life and avoid heart disease altogether. Dan Buettner teamed up with National Geographic in five longevity hotspots[30] where people reach age 100 at rates ten times greater than in the United States: Okinawa, Sardinia, Nicoya, Icaria, and among the Seventh-day Adventists in Loma Linda, California. Buettner's analysis shows that the secret is predominately plant-based diet, exercise, no smoking, family first, social engagement and a life purpose. This is very reassuring to know we are in control of our health destiny with our lifestyle choices. Since most disease processes have a multifactorial component, exercise should not be overlooked. Furthermore, the indigenous and rural populations with a low incidence of heart disease are extremely active, burning lots of calories, and virtually no one in those cultures is overweight, let alone obese. There are many studies that have shown that exercise is an independent risk factor for heart disease. In other words, those who don't exercise regularly are at higher risk.[31] One can dramatically lower the risk of heart disease by exercising regularly.[32-34]

One aspect of excellent cardiovascular health that cannot be overlooked and is the foundation of excellent health is stress reduction. Mental factors in the form of stress and emotions can contribute to high blood pressure, which can damage the heart. Stress in the form of tension, sadness, and frustration are associated with higher rates of myocardial ischemia.[35] Turbulent emotions, such as defensive-ness, anger, and hostility, have been consistently associated with stress-related blood pressure surges that can put one at risk for cardiovascular events.[36]

Since we know that early athersclerotic lesions are found in childhood, it is important to support lifestyle modification in youth to prevent coronary heart disease.[37] In sum, to live a long and healthy life, without heart disease, the following wellness plan should be followed. 1) Eat a whole-food, plant-based diet. 2) Exercise every day for about one hour. 3) Maintain a healthy weight. 4) Avoid smoking and drugs. 5) Reduce stress by daily meditation and mindfulness. 6) Take 250 mg of an algae-derived DHA/EPA supplement daily.

Pearls from Chapter 6

Cardiovascular disease is a preventable worldwide epidemic. In America, it has been the number one leading cause of death for an astounding ninety-three consecutive years and counting! The great news is heart disease is preventable and even revers-ible! It is sad and astonishing to note that in America a child by the age of ten years old has CAD with fatty streaks visible on the coronary arteries. The secret to living a long and healthy life, without heart disease, is to eat an organic whole-food, plant-based diet, rich in phytochemicals, vitamins, minerals, omega-3 fatty acids, and fiber. Also, be physically active for about one hour per day, maintain your ideal body weight, avoid smoking and drugs, and reduce stress by daily meditation and mindfulness.

CHAPTER 6 ENDNOTES

1. Yusuf S, Hawken S, Ounpuu S, et al. Effect of potentially modifiable risk factors associated with myocardial infarction in 52 countries (the INTERHEART study): case-control study. *Lancet.* 2004; 364(9438):937-952.

2. Strong JP, McGill HC Jr. The pediatric aspects of atherosclerosis. *J Atheroscler Res.*1969;9(3):251-265.

3. McMahan CA, Gidding SS, Fayad ZA. Risk scores predict atherosclerotic lesions in young people. *Arch Intern Med.* 2005;165(8):883-890.

4. Esselstyn C. *Prevent and Reverse Heart Disease.* 1st ed. New York, NY: Penguin; 2008.

5. Ornish DM, Brown SE, Scherwitz LW, et al. Can lifestyle changes reverse coronary atherosclerosis? The Lifestyle Heart Trial. *Lancet.* 1990;336:129-133. (Reprinted in Yearbook of Medicine and Yearbook of Cardiology New York: CV Mosby, 1991).

6. Reddy KS, Yusuf S. Emerging Epidemic of Cardiovascular Disease in Developing Countries. Circulation 1998;97:596-601. doi: 101161/01CIR976596.

7. Enos WF, Holmes RH, Beyer J. Coronary disease among United States soldiers killed in action in Korea; preliminary report. *J Am Med Assoc.*1953;152(12):1090-1093.

8. Heart Disease Facts. Centers for Disease Control and Prevention website. http://www.cdc.gov/heartdisease/facts.htm.

9. Heart Disease Fact Sheet. Centers for Disease Control and Prevention website. http://www.cdc.gov/dhdsp/data_statistics/fact_sheets/fs_heart_disease.htm.

10. Esselstyn CB. Updating a 12-year experience with arrest and reversal therapy for Preventing and Reversing Heart Disease coronary heart disease (an overdue requiem for palliative cardiology). *Am J Cardiol.* 1999;84(3):339-341.

11. Rimm EB, Ascherio A, Giovannucci E, Spiegelman D, Stampfer MJ, Willett WC. Vegetable, fruit, and cereal fiber intake and risk of coronary heart disease among men. *JAMA.*1996;275(6):447-451.

12. Wolk A, Manson JE, Stampfer MJ, et al. Long-term intake of dietary fiber and decreased risk of coronary heart disease among women. *JAMA.* 1999;281(21):1998.

13. Law MR, Morris JK. By how much does fruit and vegetable consumption reduce the risk of ischaemic heart disease? *Eur J Clin Nutr.* 1998;52(8)549-556.

14. Ornish DM, Brown SE, Scherwitz LW, et al. Can lifestyle changes reverse coronary atherosclerosis? The Lifestyle Heart Trial. *Lancet.* 1990;336(8708):129-133. (Reprinted in Yearbook of Medicine and Yearbook of Cardiology, New York: CV Mosby, 1991)

15. Gould KL, Ornish D, Scherwitz L, et al. Changes in myocardial perfusion abnormalities by positron emission tomography after long-term, intense risk factor modification. *JAMA.* 1995;274(11):894-901.

16. Ornish D, Scherwitz L, Billings J, et al. Intensive lifestyle changes for reversal of coronary heart disease. *JAMA.* 1998;280(23):2001-2007.

17. Ornish D. Avoiding Revascularization with Lifestyle

Changes: The Multicenter Lifestyle Demonstration Project. *Am J Cardiol.* 1998;82(10B):72T-76T.

18. Lindeberg S, Nilsson-Ehle P, Terént A. Cardiovascular risk factors in a Melanesian population apparently free from stroke and ischaemic heart disease: the Kitava study. *J Intern Med.* 1994;236(3):331-340.

19. Lindeberg, S and Vessby, B. Fatty acid composition of cholesterol esters and serum tocopherols in Melanesians apparently free from cardiovascular disease - the Kitava study. *Nutr Metab Cardiovasc Dis.* 1995;5:45-53.

20. Lindeberg S, Lundh B. Apparent absence of stroke and ischaemic heart disease in a traditional Melanesian island: a clinical study in Kitava. *J Intern Med.* 1993;233(3):269-275.

21. Thomas WA, Davies JN, O'Neal RM, Dimakulangan AA. Incidence of myocardial infarction correlated with venous and pulmonary thrombosis and embolism. A geographic study based on autopsies in Uganda, East Africa, and St. Louis, U.S.A. *Am J Cardiol.* 1960;5:41-47.

22. Shaper AG, Jones KW. Serum-cholesterol, diet, and coronary heart-disease in Africans and Asians in Uganda: 1959. *Int J Epidemiol.* 2012;41(5):1221-1225. doi: 101093/ije/dys137.

23. Bernstein AM, Willcox BJ, Tamaki H. First autopsy study of an Okinawan centenarian: absence of many age-related diseases. *J Gerontol A Biol Sci Med Sci.* 2004;59(11):1195-1199.

24. Pan A, Chen M, Chowdhury R, et al. α-Linolenic acid and risk of cardiovascular disease: a systematic review and meta-analysis. *The American Journal of Clinical Nutrition.*

2012;96(6):1262-1273. doi:103945/ajcn112044040

25. Zhao G, Etherton TD, Martin KR, West SG, Gillies PJ, Kris-Etherton PM. Dietary alpha-linolenic acid reduces inflammatory and lipid cardiovascular risk factors in hypercholesterolemic men and women. *J Nutr.* 2004;134(11):2991-2997.

26. Mozaffarian D, Wu JH. Omega-3 fatty acids and cardiovascular disease: effects on risk factors, molecular pathways, and clinical events. *J Am Coll Cardiol.* 2011;58(20):2047-2067. doi: 101016/jjacc201106063.

27. Mozaffarian D, Lemaitre RN, King IB, et al. Plasma Phospholipid Long-Chain Omega-3 Fatty Acids and Total and Cause-Specific Mortality in Older Adults: the Cardiovascular Health Study. *Annals of internal medicine.* 2013;158(7):515-525. doi:107326/0003-4819-158-7- 201304020-00003.

28. Zheng J, Huang T, Yu Y, Hu X, Yang B, Li D. Fish consumption and CHD mortality: an updated meta-analysis of seventeen cohort studies. *Public Health Nutr.* 2012;15(4):725-737. doi: 101017/S1368980011002254.

29. Kromhout D. Omega-3 fatty acids and coronary heart disease. The final verdict? *Curr Opin Lipidol.* 2012;23(6):554-559. doi: 101097/MOL0b013e328359515f.

30. Buettner D. *The Blue Zones: Lessons for Living Longer From the People Who've Lived the Longest.* 2nd ed. Washington, DC: National Geographic; 2012

31. Leon AS, Connett J, Jacobs DR Jr, Rauramaa R. Leisure-time physical activity levels and risk of coronary heart disease and death. The Multiple Risk Factor Intervention Trial. *JAMA.* 1987;258(17):2388-2395.

32. Powell KE, Thompson PD, Caspersen CJ, Kendrick JS. Physical activity and the incidence of coronary heart disease. *Annu Rev Public Health*. 1987;8:253-287.

33. Rodriguez BL, Curb JD, Burchfiel CM, et al. Physical activity and 23-year incidence of coronary heart disease morbidity and mortality among middle-aged men. The Honolulu Heart Program. *Circulation*. 1994;89(6):2540-2544.

34. Paffenbarger RS Jr, Hyde RT, Wing AL, et al The association of changes in physical-activity level and other lifestyle characteristics with mortality among men. *N Engl J Med*. 1993;328(8):538-545.

35. Gullette EC, Blumenthal JA, Babyak M. Effects of Mental Stress on Myocardial Ischemia During Daily Life. *JAMA*.1997;277(19):1521-1526. doi:101001/jama199703540430033029.

36. Grossman P, Watkins LL, Ristuccia H, Wilhelm FH. Blood pressure responses to mental stress in emotionally defensive patients with stable coronary artery disease. *Am J Cardiol*. 1997. 80(3):343–346.

37. McMahan CA, Gidding SS, Malcom GT, Tracy RE, Strong JP, McGill HC Jr; Pathobiological determinants of atherosclerosis in youth risk scores are associated with early and advanced atherosclerosis. *Pediatrics*. 2006;118(4):1447-1455.

CHAPTER SEVEN

PREVENTING AND REVERSING HYPERTENSION

It's infrequent that people are rail thin yet have high blood pressure.
—ERIC TOPOL, M.D.

If you don't know your blood pressure, it's like not knowing the value of your company.
—MEHMET OZ, M.D.

People with high blood pressure, diabetes - those are conditions brought about by lifestyle. If you change the lifestyle, those conditions will leave.
—DICK GREGORY

I HAVE A FORTY-NINE-YEAR-OLD FEMALE PATIENT who had morbid obesity, with a BMI of 47.8. She is five-foot, three-inches tall and weighed 270 pounds. The adiposity was constricting her diaphragm, and she was having trouble breathing at rest and she had hypertension, with blood pressure of 160/100. After starting her on a whole-food, plant-based diet and exercise plan she was able to lose seventy-five pounds in six months and is feeling better than ever.

High blood pressure or hypertension (HTN) is when your blood exerts excessive force on your arteries. This elevated pressure against the arterial wall leads to damage over time. Every major organ in the body has arteries that help deliver oxygenated blood and nutrients to the 10 trillion cells in your body. Over time, uncontrolled HTN leads to damaged arteries and compromises blood flow to end organs and can cause heart failure, kidney failure, stroke, blindness, heart attack, atrial fibrillation, dementia, erectile dysfunction, peripheral vascular disease, and premature death. However, if we maintain a normal blood pressure we can avoid all the previously mentioned complications of HTN. In fact, maintaining a normal blood pressure will ensure that the thousands of miles of arteries in the body remain healthy even into advanced age and all the major organs of the body will remain healthy.

According to the Center for Disease Control, one in three Americans have HTN, which is about 70 million U.S. adults.[1] The issue is that most people don't know they have HTN because most are asymptomatic. Therefore, HTN is known as the "silent killer" because many times the initial presentation is with a stroke or heart attack and at that point it may be too late. HTN can be categorized as primary or secondary. Primary HTN is also known as essential or idiopathic because modern medicine does not have a definite underlying cause and occurs in approximately 90 percent of cases. Secondary HTN is diagnosed about 10 percent of the time and has known underlying causes. Although primary HTN has no known underlying causes, there are well established risk factors.

Let's discuss some of the risk factors for high blood pressure we know from scientific data: genetics, nicotine, excess sodium intake, caffeine, excess alcohol intake, obesity or overweight, physical inactivity, vitamin D deficiency, and mental health disorders such as depression, to name a few.[2-7] Not to be overlooked, the Standard American Diet is a risk factor for HTN because of the excessive sugar, refined oils, and sodium, and mineral deficiencies such as calcium, magnesium, potassium, and zinc. Conventional medicine recommends the Dietary Approach to Stop Hypertension (DASH diet), which encourages people toward a more vegetarian diet since we have a plethora of studies showing that fruits and vegetables lower blood pressure.

An underlying cause or secondary high blood pressure should always be considered and ruled out by your doctor depending on your personal history and symptoms. Some of the causes of secondary high blood pressure include kidney disease, certain drugs such as oral contraceptives, nonsteroidal anti-inflammatory agents such as motrin and naprosyn, herbal products like ephedra, diet pills, decongestants, chronic alcohol intake, some tumors of the adrenals named pheochromocytoma, primary aldosteronism (Conn's syndrome), or Cushing's syndrome, hypothyroidism, hyperthyroidism, hyperparathyroidism, obstructive sleep apnea, acromegaly, or an abnormality of the aorta.[8] In other words, a patient should have a thorough evaluation to ensure that secondary high blood pressure is not caused by tumors, kidney disease, thyroid disease, sleep apnea, congenital narrowing of the aorta, drugs, and dietary supplements. According to the Joint National Committee (JNC) in 2013, HTN is diagnosed based upon the average of two or more properly measured readings at each of two or more clinic visits after an initial screen. The definition of HTN is as follows:

- Normal blood pressure: systolic <120 mmHg and diastolic <80 mmHg
- Prehypertension: systolic 120 to 139 mmHg or diastolic 80 to 89 mmHg
- Stage 1 hypertension: systolic 140 to 159 mmHg or diastolic 90 to 99 mmHg
- Stage 2 hypertension: systolic ≥160 or diastolic ≥100 mmHg

Once your doctor has made the diagnosis of hypertension, the usual first-line treatment is lifestyle modification. Indeed, it is ironic that although primary hypertension by definition has no known cause according the conventional paradigm, many times successful implementation of lifestyle measures cures HTN. These lifestyle measures include weight reduction, dietary sodium reduction, eating more fruits and veggies, aerobic physical activity, and limiting alcohol consumption. If these lifestyle measures do not cure your HTN then your doctor may prescribe a blood pressure pill. Also, if your initial blood pressure is too high your doctor may decide to initiate blood pressure medication along with lifestyle measures until your blood pressure is under control. This chapter will focus on how you can prevent and even reverse HTN with lifestyle choices, especially with nutrition, stress reduction and evidence-based supplementation.

An integrative holistic approach to preventing and treating HTN involves controlling psychological stress and lifestyle factors. One should also maintain an optimal body weight, perform regular aerobic exercise, eat an organic whole-food, plant-based diet, limit alcohol, avoid smoking, and have a regular meditation and mindfulness practice.

It is important to note that subjective mental factors in the form of stress and emotions can contribute to HTN. Feelings such as tension, sadness, and frustration are associated with higher rates of myocardial ischemia.[9] Turbulent emotions such as defensiveness, anger, and hostility have consistently been associated with stress-related blood pressure surges that can put one at risk for cardiovascular events.[10]

Step number one to superior health is to control stress. Modern medicine considers the cause "unknown" in up to 90 percent of cases of hypertension. In my opinion and clinical experience, the power of stress and the psychological causes of hypertension are grossly underestimated. During acute stressful situations there is a physiologic and transient rise in blood pressure, and there is no evidence that this leads to hypertension. However, chronic uncontrolled stress has been investigated and, not surprisingly, there is a significant association between chronic stress and hypertension.[11-12] It cannot be overstated, stress reduction programs, specifically meditation and mindfulness, are effective at reducing blood pressure.[13-14] Refer to chapter two of this book for effective meditation techniques to help reduce stress.

Once stress is managed effectively, the next thing to address for preventing and reversing hypertension is nutrition. There are healing compounds found in organic fruits, vegetable, grains, seeds, and nuts, that are often devoid or negligible in animal foods. These compounds include fiber, antioxidants, linoleic acid, low glycemic complex carbohydrates, minerals, and tens of thousands of phytochemicals that help reduce blood pressure. Let us explore some studies that show this association between a whole-food, plant-based diet and lower blood pressure.

A study published in 2002 from the United Kingdom found a higher prevalence of hypertension and a higher mean systolic and diastolic blood pressure among meat eaters.[15] This study analyzed more than eleven thousand British men and women aged twenty to seventy-eight for self-reported hypertension and mean blood pressure in four diet groups. The conclusion of the study was that non-meat eaters had lower blood pressure largely from differences of body mass index.

We have known for years that a vegetarian diet helps lower blood pressure. One study published in the *Lancet* in 1983 compared the effects of a lacto-ovo-vegetarian diet to an omnivorous diet in healthy normotensive subjects. After controlling for age, obesity, heart rate, weight change, and blood pressure before dietary intervention, it was found that a plant-based diet reduced systolic blood pressure by 5-6 mm Hg and diastolic blood pressure by 2-3 mm Hg. The researchers noted that the blood-pressure changes were not related to sodium or potassium intake but another unknown compound found in plants.[16]

There are thousands of named and unnamed compounds in vegetation that confer health benefits. A systematic review and meta-analysis published in 2014 in *JAMA* found the following: vegetarian diets showed a reduction in systolic BP of 4.8 mm Hg and reduction of diastolic BP of 2.2 mm Hg compared to an omnivorous diet.[17] The authors' conclusion was that a vegetarian diet should be considered as a non-pharmacologic approach at reducing blood pressure. We have a plethora of data that vegetables, either cooked or raw, help in lowering blood pressure.[18-23] One proposed mechanism is that fruits and vegetables are high in fiber whereas animal products are devoid of fiber, and increasing fiber has been associated with lowering blood pressure.[24]

There are other compounds found in plants that can help lower blood pressure. A similar study published in 2012 evaluated the effects of beetroot juice consumption on blood pressure in healthy subjects.[25] This was a double-blind, randomized, placebo-controlled trial evaluating the blood pressure of fifteen men and fifteen women after the consumption of beetroot juice, apple juice, or placebo juice. The conclusion was that the consumption of beetroot juice lowers blood pressure in men when consumed as part of a normal diet in healthy adults. The postulated mechanism for this blood pressure reduction is dietary nitrates. Interestingly, there was no effect statistically demonstrated in women.

It is estimated that 80 percent of dietary nitrates come from vegetable consumption. The vegetables with the highest nitrates content are lettuce, carrots, bok choy, beets, spinach, cabbage, celery, collard greens, leeks, broccoli, and other root vegetables. It is important not to use antibacterial mouthwash prior to ingesting dietary nitrates. There are commensal bacteria in our mouth that helps with the conversion to nitric oxide, and using commercial antibacterial mouthwash will attenuate circulating blood levels of this compound. Also, it is best to get dietary nitrate from organic whole-plant foods that will have vitamin C, polyphenols, and fatty acids that function synergistically and help prevent nitrosamines, which have been linked to cancer. I do not recommend nitrates from processed meats since the American Institute Of Cancer Research has conclusively shown a link between processed meat and cancer. Not only is there promising research that dietary nitrates help lower blood pressure, but it is also helpful for peripheral artery disease or any disease related to reduced blood flow. Undoubtedly the safest route to get dietary nitrates is through vegetable consumption.

Flaxseeds have shown impressive results in lowering of blood pressure.[26] In a recent double-blind, placebo-controlled, randomized trial, 110 total patients were given 30 grams of milled flaxseed or placebo each day for six months. After the six month intervention and controlling for weight, the flax-fed group had a 10 mm Hg lower systolic blood pressure and a 7 mm Hg lower diastolic blood pressure compared to placebo group. I have seen similar results in my clinical practice. Even more impressive was the fact that those who entered the trial with a systolic blood pressure of greater than 140 mm Hg obtained a 15 mm Hg reduction from flaxseed ingestion. The researchers concluded that four components within flaxseed may be responsible for the antihypertensive effects: omega-3 fatty acids, fiber, peptides, or a synergistic action of all four components together exert anti-inflammatory, antioxidant action, and inhibitory effect on angiotensin-converting enzyme. It is fascinating to note that these impressive effects were obtained in patients that had an average age of sixty-seven years. 75 percent or greater had hypertension and hyperlipidemia. 32 percent were diabetic. 90 percent were current or ex-smokers. One simple strategy we could implement is to consume a diet rich in organic whole foods and plants when we are young to avoid getting these chronic diseases in the first place.

Another compound that was recently found to have a statistically significant blood pressure-reducing effect is flavanol-rich cocoa products.[27] It is the flavanols, which are compounds synthesized by plants that have antioxidant activities. Flavanols increase the formation of endothelial nitric oxide, producing vasodilation thus blood pressure reduction. My recommended approach to incorporating the health-promoting effects of the cacao bean is to eat a small piece of dark chocolate with at least 70 percent cocoa several times per week. Even better, 100 percent cocoa powder can be used for smoothies, in oatmeal, or making a chocolate-flavored frozen fruit ice dessert.

I recommend getting all of one's nutrients from whole plant foods, but there are some nutritional supplements that should be considered in people who have hypertension. Studies have found vitamin C supplementation is effective at reducing blood pressure.[28] I recommend that hypertensive patients take 500 mg of vitamin C per day in consultation with a physician to monitor blood pressure. Studies show that vitamin C supplementation can lower blood pressure in subjects with normal blood pressure or elevated blood pressure. I do not recommend exceeding 1,000 mg of vitamin C regularly because of the risk of oxalate kidney stone formation for those at high risk.

There is controversy about the effectiveness of calcium supplementation on lowering blood pressure. Some research suggests that supplemental calcium can lower systolic blood pressure by up to 2.5 mm Hg.[29] However because of the weak evidence in helping with hypertension and the risk of harm I recommend against routine calcium supplementation—especially because calcium supplementation has been linked to increased risk of cardiovascular mortality. A recent study found that men, but not women, who take greater than 1,000 mg of supplemental calcium have an increased risk of death from cardiovascular disease.[30]

Vitamin D blood concentration is inversely associated with hypertension.[5] I recommend that postmenopausal women with osteoporosis take 1,200 mg of calcium and 800 I.U. of vitamin D daily. I recommend daily vitamin D of 1,000 I.U. to 3,000 I.U. depending on sun exposure, season, geographical location, age, and current blood levels.

A promising supplement in the treatment of hypertension is CoQ10. Evidence shows that coenzyme Q10 can potentially have powerful blood pressure lowering effects. It was found to lower systolic blood pressure by up to seventeen points and diastolic blood pressure by up to ten points.[31] I recommend 120 mg of coenzyme Q10 per day with food, in consultation with a physician.

Another supplement that is extremely safe to consume on a regular basis and has powerful blood pressure lowering and cholesterol lowering effects is hibiscus tea.[32] I recommend two to three cups of hibiscus tea per day. Hibiscus has abundant phytochemicals such as anthocyanins and polyphenols that have beneficial effects.

In sum, the best way to prevent and treat high blood pressure is through lifestyle. Lifestyle measures involve maintaining your optimal weight, eating an organic whole-food, plant-based diet, exercising regularly, not smoking, no drugs, and not drinking alcohol in excess. Also, a daily practice of mindfulness and meditation to control stress is crucial.

PEARLS FROM CHAPTER 7

According to the CDC about 70 million American adults have high blood pressure or about one in every three American adults. Hypertension is known as the silent killer because most people with the disease are asymptomatic. However, hypertension greatly increases the risk of heart disease and stroke. Subjective mental factors in the form of stress and emotions can contribute to HTN. Once stress is managed effectively, the next thing to address for preventing and reversing hypertension is nutrition. There are healing compounds found in organic fruits, vegetables, grains, seeds, and nuts, but are often devoid or negligible in animal foods. These compounds include fiber, antioxidants, linoleic acid, low glycemic complex carbohydrates, minerals, and tens of thousands of phytochemicals that help reduce blood pressure. The most effective strategy to prevent and reverse hypertension is by lifestyle measures that involve maintaining your optimal weight, eating an organic whole-food, plant-based diet, exercising regularly, not smoking, no drugs, and not drinking alcohol in excess. Hypertensive patients, in consultation with a physician, should consider the following foods and supplements as part of their daily diet: beets, flaxseeds, cocoa, coenzyme Q10, vitamin C, and hibiscus tea.

CHAPTER 7 ENDNOTES

1. High Blood Pressure. Centers for Disease Control and Prevention. http://www.cdc.gov/bloodpressure/.

2. Forman JP, Stampfer MJ, Curhan GC. Diet and lifestyle risk factors associated with incident hypertension in women. *JAMA*. 2009;302(4):401-411.

3. Meng L, Chen D, Yang Y, Zheng Y, Hui R. Depression increases the risk of hypertension incidence: a meta-analysis of prospective cohort studies. *J Hypertens*. 2012;30(5):842-851.

4. Carnethon MR, Evans NS, Church TS, et al. Joint associations of physical activity and aerobic fitness on the development of incident hypertension: coronary artery risk development in young adults. *Hypertension*. 2010;56(1):49-55.

5. Burgaz A, Orsini N, Larsson SC, Wolk A. Blood 25-hydroxyvitamin D concentration and hypertension: a meta-analysis. *J Hypertens*. 2011;29(4):636-645.

6. He FJ, MacGregor GA. Salt, blood pressure and cardio-vascular diseases. *Curr Opin Cardiol*. 2007;22(4):298-305.

7. Wang NY, Young JH, Meoni LA, Ford DE, Erlinger TP, Klag MJ. Blood pressure change and risk of hypertension associated with parental hypertension: the Johns Hopkins Precursors Study. *Arch Intern Med*. 2008;168(6):643-648.

8. Viera A, Neutze D. Diagnosis of Secondary Hypertension: An Age-Based Approach. *Am Fam Physician*. 2010;82(12):1471-1478.

9. Gullette EC, Blumenthal JA, Babyak M, et al. Effects of Mental Stress on Myocardial Ischemia During Daily Life. *JAMA*.1997;277(19):1521-1526. doi:101001/ *JAMA*199703540430033029.

10. Grossman P, Watkins LL, Ristuccia H, Wilhelm FH. Blood pressure responses to mental stress in emotionally defensive patients with stable coronary artery disease. *Am J Cardiol*. 1997;80(3):343–346.

11. Spruill TM. Chronic Psychosocial Stress and Hypertension. *Curr Hypertens Rep*. 2010;12(1):10-16. doi:101007/ s11906-009-0084-8.

12. Sparrenberger F, Cichelero FT, Ascoli AM, et al. Does psychosocial stress cause hypertension? A systematic review of observational studies. *J Hum Hypertens*. 2009;23(1):12–19. doi:101038/jhh200874.

13. Rainforth MV, Schneider RH, Nidich SI, Gaylord-King C, Salerno JW, Anderson JW. Stress Reduction Programs in Patients with Elevated Blood Pressure: A Sys-

tematic Review and Meta-analysis. *Curr Hypertens Rep.* 2007;9(6):520-528.

14. Jain S, Shapiro SL, Swanick S, et al. A randomized controlled trial of mindfulness meditation versus relaxation training: effects on distress, positive states of mind, rumination, and distraction. *Ann Behav Med.* 2007;33(1):11-21.

15. Appleby PN, Davey GK, Key TJ. Hypertension and blood pressure among meat eaters, fish eaters, vegetarians and vegans in EPIC–Oxford. *Public Health Nutr.* 2002;5(5):645-654. doi:101079/PHN2002332.

16. Rouse IL, Beilin LJ, Armstrong BK, Vandongen R. Blood-pressure-lowering effect of a vegetarian diet: controlled trial in normotensive subjects. *Lancet.* 1983; 1(8314-8315): 5–10.

17. Yokoyama Y, Nishimura K, Barnard ND, et al. Vegetarian diets and blood pressure: a meta-analysis. *JAMA Intern Med.* 2014;174(4):577-587. doi:101001/jamainternmed201314547.

18. Chan Q, Stamler J, Brown IJ, et al. Relations of raw and cooked vegetable consumption to blood pressure: the INTERMAP. *J Hum Hypertens.* 2013;28(6):353-359. doi:101038/jhh2013115.

19. Armstrong B, van Merwyk AJ, Coates H. Blood pressure in Seventh-day Adventist vegetarians. *Am J Epidemiol.* 1977;105(5):444–449.

20. Margetts BM, Beilin LJ, Vandongen R, Armstrong BK. Vegetarian diet in mild hypertension: a randomised controlled trial. *Br Med J* (Clin Res Ed). 1986;293(6560):1468-1471.

21. Nunez-Cordoba JM, Alonso A, Beunza JJ, Palma S,

Gomez-Gracia E, Martinez-Gonzalez MA. Role of vegetables and fruits in Mediterranean diets to prevent hypertension. *Eur J Clin Nutr.* 2009;63(5):605–612.

22. Wang L, Manson JE, Gaziano JM, Buring JE, Sesso HD. Fruit and vegetable intake and the risk of hypertension in middle-aged and older women. *Am J Hypertens.* 2012; 25(2):180–189.

23. Pettersen BJ, Anousheh R, Fn J, Jaceldo-Siegl K, Fraser GE. Vegetarian diets and blood pressure among white subjects: results from the Adventist Health Study-2 (AHS-2). *Public Health Nutr.* 2012;15(10):1909-1916.

24. Streppel MT, Arends LR, van't Veer P, Grobbee DE, Geleijnse JM. Dietary fiber and blood pressure: a meta-analysis of randomized placebo-controlled trials. *Arch Intern Med.* 2005;165(2):150-156.

25. Coles LT, Clifton PM. Effect of beetroot juice on lowering blood pressure in free-living, disease-free adults: a randomized, placebo-controlled trial. *Nutr J.* 2012;11:106. doi:101186/1475-2891-11-106.

26. Rodriguez-Leyva D, Weighell W, Edel AL, et al. Potent antihypertensive action of dietary flaxseed in hypertensive patients. *Hypertension.* 2013;62(6):1081-1089. doi: 101161/HYPERTENSIONAHA11302094.

27. Ried K, Sullivan TR, Fakler P, Frank OR, Stocks NP. Effect of cocoa on blood pressure. *Cochrane Database Syst Rev.* 2012;8:CD008893. doi: 101002/14651858.CD008893pub2.

28. Juraschek SP, Guallar E, Appel LJ, Miller ER. Effects of vitamin C supplementation on blood pressure: a meta-analysis of randomized controlled trials. *Am J Clin Nutr.* 2012;95(5):1079-1088. doi:10.3945/ajcn111027995.

29. Dickinson HO, Nicolson DJ, Cook JV, et al. Calcium supplementation for the management of primary hypertension in adults. *Cochrane Database Syst Rev.* 2006;(2):CD004639.

30. Xiao Q, Murphy RA, Houston DK, Harris TB, Chow WH, Park Y. Dietary and supplemental calcium intakes in relation to mortality from cardiovascular diseases in the NIH-AARP Diet and Health Study. *JAMA Intern Med.* 2013;173(8):639-646. doi:101001/jamainternmed20133283.

31. Rosenfeldt FL, Haas SJ, Krum H, Hadj A, Ng K, Leong JY, Watts GF. Coenzyme Q10 in the treatment of hypertension: a meta-analysis of the clinical trials. *J Hum Hypertens.* 2007;21(4):297-306.

32. Hopkins AL, Lamm MG, Funk J, Ritenbaugh C. *Hibiscus sabdariffa* L. in the treatment of hypertension and hyperlipidemia: a comprehensive review of animal and human studies. *Fitoterapia.* 2013;85:84-94. doi:101016/j fitote201301003.

CHAPTER EIGHT

PREVENTING AND REVERSING GASTROINTESTINAL DISEASE

We are inhabited by as many as ten thousand bacterial species; those cells outnumber those which we consider our own by ten to one, and weigh, all told, about three pounds--the same as our brain. Together, they are referred to as our microbiome---and they play such a crucial role in our lives that scientists like [Martin J.] Blaser have begun to reconsider what it means to be human.

—MICHAEL SPECTER

Warren Buffet told me once and he said always follow your gut. When you have that gut feeling, you have to go with don't go back on it.

—LEBRON JAMES

DEBBIE IS A THIRTY-FIVE-YEAR-OLD SINGLE MOM who works full time. She has enormous stress at work and the challenges of being a single parent are overwhelming. She presented to my office with fatigue, mental fogginess, bloating, gas pain, acid reflux, alternating bouts of diarrhea and constipation, and depressed mood. She had seen several gastroenterologists and had an endoscopy, colonoscopy, lab work including CBC, CMP, ESR, stool cultures and everything came back normal. She was diagnosed with irritable bowel syndrome and placed on medication. She was not tolerating the side effects of the pharmaceuticals and wanted an integrative holistic approach to her care. After carefully reviewing her case, I suggested we get a comprehensive gastrointestinal stool analysis. This stool analysis is a functional medicine test that uses polymerase chain reaction (PCR) amplification techniques to test the DNA and RNA to evaluate the diversity and abundance of the microbiome. It also tests for any parasites or pathogens present, inflammation, digestive insufficiencies or imbalances. Upon review of my patient's results, she had small intestine bacterial overgrowth (SIBO), and several pathogenic strains of bacteria and candida overgrowth. I recommended plant-based digestive enzymes, prebiotics, increase in resistant starches and fiber, and peppermint gel caps three times per day with meals. I also recommended she focus on a low glycemic, whole-food, plant-based diet and a daily fifteen-minute breathing meditation to help control stress. On follow-up visits, Debbie is doing better than she has done in years.

The human gastrointestinal (GI) tract is amazing! It is astonishing to think that the human body contains more than ten times as many microbes in our GI tract than human cells. In other words, the human body contains 10 trillion cells, and our GI tract has 100 trillion microbes! The surface area of humans' GI tract has been calculated by some to be up to 300 square meters. That's larger than a tennis court. The length of the GI tract from mouth to anus is about nine meters in an average adult, which is about thirty feet. Classically, the GI tract was viewed more as a mechanical organ in charge of digestion and absorption of food. Emerging research has shown us the GI tract is much more. The GI tract has neuronal cells, endocrine cells, and immune cells. It is our second brain, technically known as the enteric nervous system. Our GI tract contains 100 million neurons, which is more than our peripheral nervous system and our spinal cord, and 95 percent of the body's serotonin is found in our gut! Because of this extensive neuronal connection between our gut and our brain, mental stress can directly be felt in our GI tract as butterflies in the stomach--a gut reaction. Our gut is home to 70-80 percent of our immune system and there are more than twenty identified hormones produced by our GI tract. Once we appreciate the complexity of the GI tract, we can see how stress can directly negatively impact and affect our guts neurons, hormones, and immune cells and lead to disease.

Studies have shown that mindfulness based stress reduction can decrease symptoms of IBS.[1] It is important to control stress by setting boundaries and having a healthy work life balance. Uncontrolled stress can lead to overextending oneself and becoming all consumed with work. We know that work exhaustion can lead to premature biological aging by shortening telomere length over time. But we also know that psychological stress can interfere with healthy biological rhythms and sleep-wake cycles. It is common for stress to lead to restlessness and insomnia. Not sleeping leads to having the late-night munchies and eating late into the night, which is very harmful to the body. Over time, this habit can lead to disease because the body does not have adequate time to detox and cleanse itself with an overnight fast. And more importantly, stress can lead to poor decision-making and eating the wrong foods.

In today's society, humans are consuming toxic food for the body. Unfortunately, there is a pervasive American myth: "Real men eat steak." At football games, barbeques, potlucks, etc., it is blasphemy if you don't find some red meat. Red meat and processed meat consumption has been associated with increased death from cancer, heart disease, and all cause mortality, according to an NIH-AARP cohort study of 1/2 million people.[2] Also, a study published in March 2012 had a similar finding showing an association between red meat consumption and higher risk of dying from heart disease, cancer, and all-cause mortality.[3] Dr. Frank Hu, Professor of Nutrition at Harvard states: "This study provides clear evidence that regular consumption of red meat, especially processed meat, contributes substantially to premature death." Regrettably, the US Dietary Guidelines have not received the memo that red meat is toxic. They still recommend two to three servings of red meat in a 2,000 calorie diet as a good protein source. Even more unfortunate, millions of Americans continue eating an average of 110 pounds of red meat per year. Experts at the American Institute for Cancer Research (AICR) suggest that Americans limit or avoid red meat consumption since the link between red meat and colon cancer is now convincing. Furthermore, "The meat-and-potatoes mindset is slowly killing us," said AICR Nutrition Advisor Karen Collins, MS, RD. "We need to break ourselves of the notion that we need a hunk of red meat at every meal."

In October 2015, the World Health Organization's International Agency for Research on Cancer (IARC) classified high consumption of processed meat in Group 1, which assigns it the same cancer risk as tobacco smoke. Red meat is classified in Group 2A, "probably carcinogenic to humans," just as the pesticide glyphosphate.[4] In general, we have many decades of scientific data that shows a link between meat consumption and colon cancer. Colon cancer is the second leading cause of cancer death in America, in both men and women, behind only lung cancer. The well-established risk factors for developing colon cancer include genetics, family history, inflammatory bowel disease, obesity, diabetes, alcohol, and cigarette smoking. Lifestyle habits that are associated with protecting against colon cancer include physical activity, diets high in fruits and vegetables, and diets rich in folate, calcium, magnesium, and vitamin D. One risk factor that has been clearly linked with colon cancer is meat consumption.

There is epidemiological evidence that per capita meat consumption is correlated with bowel cancer deaths.[5] For example, Japanese immigrants who adopt a Standard American Diet (SAD) have a five-fold increased incidence of colon cancer.[6] Traditionally, Asian diets that consume a high percentage of plants have lower rates of cancer and this is consistent with the current literature that vegetarian diets are protective against cancer.[7] The highest incidences of colorectal cancer seen in the world are in the United States, Canada, and New Zealand. There is an impressive twenty-five-fold increase in the incidences of colon cancer in industrialized countries versus developing countries. However, the incidences of colon cancer are rapidly increasing in developing countries as well. Sadly, it takes only one generation to adopt a toxic American diet to greatly increase the risk of colon cancer. If you live in America, there is something that one can do to dramatically lower the risk of colon cancer as demonstrated by the following study published in 2015. The Adventist Health Study 2 found that vegetarian diets have much lower incidences of colorectal cancers.[8] On the other hand, consumption of red meat and processed meat, after controlling for confounders such as weight and smoking, was found to increase the risk of colon cancer.[9,10] Other studies have corroborated the association between the high consumption of red meat and processed meat and colorectal cancer but have found an inverse relationship with fish consumption.[11]

Although there seems to be an overwhelming body of scientific literature supporting the association between red meat consumption and colon cancer, there is considerable debate as to the proposed mechanism. A recent study suggests that that the mechanism is related to heme iron, nitrate/nitrite, and heterocyclic amines.[12] There are, however, other mechanisms to consider for the development of colon cancer.

The reader may wonder, "What is the connection? Why does red meat engender a higher risk of colon cancer?" The average weight of the American colon may hold the clue. The average American has ten to twenty-five pounds of fecal matter in his or her colon on autopsy. This does not have to be the case. The process of putrefaction, or decomposition of dead animals producing foul smelling stench, should not occur in the human GI tract. Putrefaction in the human bowel is not normal and this alters and increases the bacterial load in the GI tract. Studies have shown that when the microflora is altered, you get an increase in bacterial beta-glucuronidase, nitroreductase, azoreductase, and steroid 7-alpha-dehydroxylase activities. These effects happen in humans consuming a high-beef or low-fiber animal diet. Could the secret lie in the amount of fiber in the diet?

There is considerable interest and controversy on dietary fiber's link to colon cancer. Many studies have shown an association between increased dietary fiber in food and protection against colorectal cancer.[13-17] In fact, some studies suggest that by increasing dietary fiber by ten grams per day there is a reduction of colon cancer by 10 percent.[14] However, there are other studies showing no association between fiber and colon cancer.[18-21] So what is an individual to do amidst all this confusion about diet? One day it's good for you and the next day a big news story breaks stating that dietary fiber is not associated with colon cancer. I say, when it comes to food, the whole food is greater than the sum of its parts. In May 2015, in the *JAMA Internal Medicine*, nearly 100,000 subjects were examined. It was concluded that vegetarians had a lower overall incidence of colon cancer.[22] This study showed an impressive 20 percent reduction in risk of colon cancer with a vegetarian dietary pattern compared to a non-vegetarian pattern. As we have seen there are many mixed results when considering dietary fiber and colon cancer. However, when considering plant versus animal consumption, the results are clear.

Let's consider a fascinating study of African Americans compared to Native Africans. We know that the incidence of colon cancer in African Americans is dramatically higher than in Native Africans, but why? A recent study suggests that African

Americans have dramatically higher colon cancer risk because of higher dietary intake of animal products.[23] Even though both populations had the same fiber intake, because of the higher consumption of meat, saturated fat, and cholesterol, there was a high rate of colon cell proliferation and bacterial dysbiosis in African Americans. One possible explanation is that meat protein leads to colon mucosal injury by promoting "bad" bacteria.[24] It promotes sulfur-reducing bacteria, which engenders a foul odor and impairs cytochrome oxidase, colon tissue health, mucus formation, and DNA methylation. Those are just details. To translate it into simple English, I shall quote the famous saying from Eastern mystics: "Don't let your stomach be a graveyard for animals." This can lead to intestinal dysbiosis, leaky gut syndrome, SIBO (small intestinal bacterial overgrowth), or IBS (irritable bowel syndrome).

The toxic Standard American Diet leads to intestinal dysbiosis. The increase and alteration of the bacterial flora leads to the release of toxins and damages the delicate intestinal mucosa leading to a whole host of disease processes. This intestinal dysbiosis will manifest as a myriad of nonspecific symptoms including bloating, flatulence, fatigue, abdominal pain, loose stool, dyspepsia, dermatitis, IBS, arthritis, malabsorption, and weight loss or failure to gain weight in children. "Leaky gut" is a relatively new condition that is still not accepted in conventional medicine, but is fully recognized as a diagnosis in integrative medicine. In fact, there have been several studies examining the pathophysiology of intestinal permeability.[25-27] "Leaky gut" can lead to increased inflammatory cytokine production and increased inflammation that may lead to systemic disease. Again, conventional medicine is only in its rudimentary stages of understanding this condition so they attempt to diagnosis SIBO (small intestine bacterial overgrowth) with such drastic measures as a small bowel biopsy. Or they may use jejunal aspirate, a d-xylose breath test, or a breath hydrogen analysis for the diagnosis of SIBO.[28]However, a simpler and more humane way to assess for the integrity of intestinal permeability is by performing the standardized lactulose-mannitol test. The patient drinks a sugar solution, and then the ratio of these sugars are examined in the urine six hours later to assess intestinal permeability. Again, it is noted that increased intestinal permeability is linked with many diseases such as inflammatory bowel disease, asthma, diabetes, inflammatory arthritis, scleroderma, fibromyalgia, chronic myofascial pain, eczema, chronic fatigue, psychiatric disease, etc. The most important thing is identifying the underlying cause of intestinal dysbiosis. We must consider antibiotic use and narcotic use, which could lead to decreased transit time and narcotic bowel syndrome. But most importantly, one should closely examine foods consumed: are they organic, free of genetically modified organisms (GMOs), free of bovine growth hormone (BGH), high in fiber, predominantly plant based, ruling out food allergies and intolerances, etc.? Once the offending agent is identified and removed, then healthy prebiotics and probiotics should be introduced. The anti-inflammatory and immunomodulatory effects of probiotics provide the basis for therapeutic intervention. Clearly, the design of the human GI tract was not meant to handle meat, which alters the natural homeostasis of our endogenous GI flora. Let's explore why.

Children provide the perfect template for how many bowel movements adults should have. Most children have not lived long enough to carry the toxic fecal burden that most adults have. If you observe a child, many times when they take their first bite at dinner, they run to the bathroom to "poop." This phenomenon occurs because the first bite stimulated the gastrocolic reflex, which gives the urge to defecate. Why does this happen? The answer lies in the intelligent design of the body. Before ingesting more food, one should be sure to have fully digested and evacuated your previous meal, according ancient yogic wisdom. I see many patients who continue to eat breakfast, lunch, and dinner while completely disregarding colonic wellbeing and without having a bowel movement for days or weeks! Where is all that food going? It's no wonder that adults walk around feeling bloated, tired, sluggish, full, suffering with acid reflux, constipation, obesity, and generally feeling unhealthy. In contrast, children usually only eat when they are hungry and have an incredible zest for life and vitality.

Another pearl from the ancient sages is to chew food at least fifty times. The associated saying is drink your solids and eat your liquids, which prevents overeating and enhances digestion by the release of ghrelin and leptin. Also, when sitting for a meal the West has the worst possible position, i.e., sitting in a chair. This posture does not enhance digestion, but rather delays it. The optimal sitting position for eating is used in Eastern cultures: sitting on their knees with heels on sitting bone, which is called thunderbolt pose. It is said that if you sit in this position for thirty minutes after a meal you can eat another entire full meal. Please do not try this at home. I am not encouraging you to eat duplicate dinners.

Not only is how you sit while eating a meal important, but the way you sit while having a bowel movement is important. The optimal position for defecation for full evacuation is not sitting on toilet. Squatting is much more efficacious and conducive to a full evacuation. This position has been recommended in Ayurvedic medicine for thousands of years, along with a daily colon cleanse by having three bowel movements per day and weekly fasting to help detox the body. All of these measures were preventative and helped the GI tract rest and allowed for our healthy good bacteria to thrive, unlike what most Americans do today.

There is a war going on in your bowels: good bacteria versus bad bacteria! Animal products give the bad bacteria more troops, i.e., bacterial overgrowth, which leads to putrefaction, toxic waste, increase inflammatory cytokines, increased intestinal permeability, and potential lethal mutations. This is an epic battle! When you eat organic fruits and veggies, you get a daily colon cleanse, and the good friendly symbiotic bacteria are winning the battle. Plant foods provide the right fuel for your microbiome and offer the proper prebiotics and probiotics for proper GI health.

The best medicine for gastrointestinal health is eating a whole-food, plant-based diet, avoiding animal products, exercising for one hour everyday, avoiding excessive alcohol, not smoking, maintaining your ideal body weight, and controlling stress.

Pearls from Chapter 8

The GI tract is an amazing organ that houses neuronal, endocrine, and immune cells. It is our second brain, technically known as the enteric nervous system. Our GI tract contains 100 million neurons and 95 percent of the body's serotonin is found in our gut! Because of this extensive neuronal connection between our gut and our brain, mental stress can be felt directly in our GI tract as butterflies in the stomach or a gut feeling. Mental stress can negatively impact our guts neurons, hormones, and immune cells and lead to disease. Stress reduction is crucial for GI health. Also, eating an organic whole-food, plant-based diet leads to a healthy microbiome. Animal products lead to putrefaction, toxic waste, increase inflammatory cytokines, increased intestinal permeability, and potential lethal mutations. This leads to intestinal dysbiosis, SIBO, IBS, leaky gut, and increased risk of colon cancer.

Chapter 8 Endnotes

1. Zernicke KA, Campbell TS, Blustein PK, et al. Mindfulness-based stress reduction for the treatment of irritable bowel syndrome symptoms: a randomized wait-list controlled trial. *Int J Behav Med*. 2013;20(3):385-396. doi: 101007/s12529-012-9241-6.

2. Sinha R, Cross AJ, Graubard BI, Leitzmann MF, Schatzkin A. Meat intake and mortality: a prospective study of over half a million people. *Arch Intern Med*. 2009;169(6):562-571. doi:101001/archinternmed20096.

3. Pan A, Sun Q, Bernstein AM, et al. Red Meat Consumption and Mortality: Results From 2 Prospective Cohort Studies. *Arch Intern Med*. 2012;172(7):555-563. doi:101001/archinternmed20112287.

4. Consumption of red meat and processed meat, *IARC Monographs*. 2015;Vol 114.

5. Howell MA. Factor Analysis of International Cancer Mortality Data and per capita Food Consumption. *Br J Cancer*. 1974;29(4):328-336.

6. Kolonel LN, Hinds MW, and Hankin JH. Cancer patterns

among migrant and native-born Japanese in Hawaii in relation to smoking, drinking, and dietary habits. In: Gelboin H.V. et al., eds. Genetic and environmental factors in experimental and human cancer. Tokyo: Japan Sci Soc Press.1980:327-340.

7. Lanou AJ, Svenson B. Reduced cancer risk in vegetarians: an analysis of recent reports. *Cancer Manag Res*. 2011;3:1-8. doi:102147/CMRS6910.

8. Orlich MJ, Singh PN, Sabaté J, et al. Vegetarian Dietary Patterns and the Risk of Colorectal Cancers. *JAMA Intern Med*. 2015;175(5):767-776. doi:101001/jamainternmed201559.

9. Chao A, Thun MJ, Connell CJ, et al. Meat Consumption and Risk of Colorectal Cancer. *JAMA*. 2005;293(2):172-182 doi:101001/jama2932172.

10. Chan DS, Lau R, Aune D, et al. Red and Processed Meat and Colorectal Cancer Incidence: Meta-Analysis of Prospective Studies. *PLoS ONE*. 2011;6(6):e20456. doi:101371/journalpone0020456.

11. Norat T, Bingham S, Ferrari P, et al. Meat, fish, and colorectal cancer risk: the European Prospective Investigation into cancer and nutrition. *J Natl Cancer Inst*. 2005;97(12):906-916. doi:101093/jnci/dji164.

12. Cross AJ, Ferrucci LM, Risch A, et al. A large prospective study of meat consumption and colorectal cancer risk: an investigation of potential mechanisms underlying this association. *Cancer res*. 2010;70(6):2406-2414. doi:101158/0008-5472CAN-09-3929.

13. Bingham SA, Day NE, Luben R, et al. Dietary fibre in food and protection against colorectal cancer in

the European Prospective Investigation into Cancer and Nutrition (EPIC): an observational study. *Lancet.* 2003;361(9368):1496-1501.

14. Aune, D, Chan, DS, Lau, R, et al. Dietary fibre, whole grains, and risk of colorectal cancer: Preventing and Reversing Gastrointestinal Disease systematic review and dose-response meta-analysis of prospective studies. *BMJ.* 2011;343: d6617.

15. Larsson SC, Giovannucci E, Bergkvist L, Wolk A. Whole grain consumption and risk of colorectal cancer: a population-based cohort of 60,000 women. *Br J Cancer.* 2005;92(9):1803-1807. doi:101038/sjbjc6602543.

16. Howe GR, Benito E, Castelleto R, et al. Dietary intake of fiber and decreased risk of cancers of the colon and rectum: evidence from the combined analysis of 13 case-control studies. *J Natl Cancer Inst.* 1992;84(24):1887-1896.

17. Trock B, Lanza E, Greenwald P. Dietary fiber, vegetables, and colon cancer: critical review and meta-analyses of the epidemiologic evidence. *J Natl Cancer Inst.* 1990;82(8):650-661.

18. Fuchs CS, Giovannucci EL, Colditz GA, et al. Dietary fiber and the risk of colorectal cancer and adenoma in women. *N Engl J Med.* 1999;340(3):169-176.

19. Schatzkin A, Lanza E, Corle D et al. Lack of effect of a low-fat, high-fiber diet on the recurrence of colorectal adenomas Polyp Prevention Trial Study Group. *N Engl J Med.* 2000;342(16):1149-1155.

20. Alberts DS, Martínez ME, Roe DJ. Lack of effect of a high-fiber cereal supplement on the recurrence of colorectal adenomas Phoenix Colon Cancer Prevention Physicians'

Network. *N Engl J Med.* 2000;342(16):1156-1162.

21. Park Y, Hunter DJ, Spiegelman D, et al. Dietary Fiber. Intake and Risk of Colorectal Cancer: A Pooled Analysis of Prospective Cohort Studies. *JAMA.* 2005;294(22):2849-2857. doi:101001/jama294222849.

22. Orlich MJ, Singh PN, Sabaté J, et al. Vegetarian Dietary Patterns and the Risk of Colorectal Cancers. *JAMA Intern Med.* 2015;175(5):767-776. doi:101001/jamainternmed201559.

23. O'Keefe SJ, Chung D, Mahmoud N et al. Why do African Americans get more colon cancer than Native Africans? *J Nutr.* 2007;137(1 suppl):S175-182.

24. Ou J, Carbonero F, Zoetendal EG, et al. Diet, microbiota, and microbial metabolites in colon cancer risk in rural Africans and African Americans. *Am J Clin Nutr.* 2013;98(1):111-120. doi: 103945/ajcn112056689.

25. Baumgart DC, Dignass AU. Intestinal barrier function. *Curr Opin Clin Nutr Metab Care.* 2002;5(6):685-694.

26. Clayburgh DR, Shen L, Turner JR. A porous defense: the leaky epithelial barrier in intestinal disease. *Lab Invest.* 2004;84(3):282-291.

27. DeMeo MT, Mutlu EA, Keshavarzian A, Tobin MC. Intestinal permeation and gastrointestinal disease. *J Clin Gastroenterol.* 2002;34(4):385-396.

28. DiBaise JK. Nutritional consequences of small bacterial overgrowth. *Pract Gastroenterol.* 2008;69:22-25.

CHAPTER NINE

Dangers and Benefits of Supplements

Let food be thy medicine and medicine be thy food.
—Hippocrates

If we could give every individual the right amount of nourishment and exercise, not too little and not too much, we would have found the safest way to health.
—Hippocrates

Janice is a forty-four-year-old female with chronic medical problems including fatigue, gait disturbance, migraines, vertigo, and neuropathy. She had seen several specialists and no diagnosis had been found to explain her symptoms. She came to me for help. On her first visit I reviewed the eighteen different supplements she was taking and realized she was taking megadoses of vitamin B6, approximately 10,000 percent the recommended daily dose. She told me she was taking it to help her stress. When I checked her blood levels of vitamin B6, they were excessively high in the toxicity zone, and this dangerous amount of vitamin B6 was causing most of her symptoms. I adjusted her supplement list to only four that her body needs, and the rest she could obtain from a healthy plant-based diet. Her symptoms resolved and she felt the best she had in years.

Ideally, one would get all the essential vitamins, minerals, and phytochemicals from the foods we eat. As Hippocrates noted several millennia ago, food is medicine. However, with changing times and the evolution of our planet, we cannot solely rely on foods for optimal health and longevity.

A person does not need to take any supplements as long as he or she lives in a tropical paradise with rich soil, is retired without any stress, and cooks and prepares every meal from the organic garden that is burgeoning with fruits and vegetables. How many of us are living that way? If you are like most people, with a full-time job, a family, a social life, and are often eating on the run, then you will need to take a supplement to avoid deficiency.

A recent article titled "Enough Is Enough: Stop Wasting Money on Vitamin and Mineral Supplements" suggested consumers should stop taking vitamins.[1] The study is flawed because: 1) Subjects were using synthetic commercial multivitamins that I don't recommend. 2) Most of these subjects were on the SAD (Standard American Diet), so a multivitamin was not going to make a difference anyway. I recommend a whole-food based supplement with no synthetic vitamins and NO EXCESSIVE vitamin A, C, E, D, beta carotene, or vitamin B6, which have all been linked to toxicity in excessive amounts.

Finally, a whole-food, low glycemic, plant-based diet will give all the micronutrients necessary for health. For most, a whole-food based multivitamin, Vitamin D, Vitamin B12, and a DHA/EPA supplement are important in order to avoid any nutritional deficiency and are a safety net, not a substitute for a healthy diet!

The traditional teaching given to all medical students is that digestion begins in the mouth with mastication and the food bolus being saturated and broken down with salivary enzymes. Actually, the digestion of food begins before that, when we make a conscious decision that we are going to eat. First, are we truly hungry as we prepare to make our meal, or are we a slave to our watches? Second, are we choosing the foods that are nutrient dense, low glycemic, rich in phytochemicals, and low calorie? I argue that these are the first stages of digestion: it begins with our own conscious decision of whether our body is ready to eat that next meal. If indeed we decide what we should eat, we must select foods rich in vitamins, minerals and phytochemicals, and high in antioxidants. In the hectic pace of modern life running hither and thither, many times people feel forced to eat poor quality meals on the run that are detrimental to health. Realize that even in our fast-paced society, we have a choice. Swami Satchitananda once said that if you are hungry and confronted with the choice of eating an unhealthy meal to quench your hunger or skip your meal, then the latter is preferable. Skipping a meal and fasting is not only preferable in this scenario, but it can confer health benefits.[2] What is the worst that can happen? You may feel a little transient hunger but you won't be bombarding your system with toxic food stuff, so occasional fasting is a much healthier option. Research has shown that even one unhealthy meal can cause inflammation and damage to the lining of the arteries.[3] We also know that foods from the plant kingdom are loaded with a plethora of healing nutrients.

The American Cancer Society, after reviewing thousands of articles, has determined that not only are smoking and obesity risk factors for cancer, but eating red meat is a known risk factor for cancer as well. Moreover, it does not matter if the meat comes from grass-fed beef or grain-fed beef. The point is, meat does not belong in the human body. The myth that meat offers you some special kind of protein or some special kind of fatty acid has been thoroughly debunked. If you want the best, most bio-available protein source that is the easiest for your body to assimilate, then eat human flesh. Or, how about eating dog meat that is lean and high in protein? Of course, I do not recommend that, and I am sure none of you have an appetite for human flesh or dog meat. Let's briefly explore the great myths of grass-fed beef, protein, and diet fads.

Does anyone eat grass-fed beef and consider this red meat healthier and rich in omega-3s? Well,

I am here to tell you that grass-fed beef is toxic to the human body and even more toxic to the planet. As an example, a four ounce grass-fed hamburger will give you about 88 mg of omega-3 fatty acids, but it still has unhealthy saturated fats, cholesterol, and caloric density. Compare this to one tablespoon of flax seeds which gives you a grand total of 2,338 mg of omega-3 fatty acids. That's almost thirty times more than what the hamburger gives you, and it does not have any saturated fats and cholesterol and has many healthful phytochemicals! Also, which has more protein, beef or kale? Well, the protein content of 100 calories of beef versus a 100 calories of kale is very revealing. In 100 calories of kale you get 6.6 grams of protein and in 100 calories of cooked beef about nine grams of protein. That is not a significant difference. But the nutritional profile difference is very significant! So, 100 calories of kale with one tablespoon of flax provides more phyto-nutrients and complete protein than 100 calories of beef without the harmful effects.

Overall, plants are better sources of nutrients than animal products. In this chapter, I will explore some of the key nutrients and what food sources they are obtained from and key supplements for optimal health and longevity. For each nutrient or key supplement, I will briefly discuss the basics, plant sources, symptoms of deficiency, symptoms of excess, and whether or not I recommend routine supplementation. Certainly, these general statements do not constitute medical advice. Please discuss a plan with your doctor before starting or altering your supplement plan.

Vitamin A

There are more than 600 known carotenoids, which are organic compounds found in plants, better known as Vitamin A (Carotenoids). Humans are not capable of synthesizing carotenoids and must obtain them through the diet. Interestingly, vitamin A from animal sources and supplements is pre-formed, also known as retinol, and is associated with toxicity if taken in excess, because it is fat soluble and the body does not have a way to get rid of it. Symptoms associated with excessive vitamin A are headaches, nausea, dizziness, increased intracranial pressure, liver failure, coma, even death. However, the vitamin A precursor found in plants, known as beta-carotene, is not associated with toxicity even in massive doses. For example, eating too many carrots can lead to carotenodermia, a benign, reversible condition where the skin becomes yellow-orange. A deficiency of vitamin A can lead to a impaired immunity, weak bones, night blindness, leukoplakia, and hyperkeratosis. Patients with hypothyroidism, oral contraceptive pill use, and a history of alcoholism are at risk of deficiency. My favorite sources of beta-carotene are sweet potatoes, carrots, spinach, broccoli, kale, and butternut squash. I do not recommend supplementation with preformed vitamin A because of the known toxic effects. Furthermore, even supplementation with beta-carotene, which is harmless when eaten in foods, has been associated with an increased risk of lung cancer, cardiovascular disease, and increased risk of mortality. [4-6] I do not recommend routine supplementation with vitamin A or beta-carotene.

Vitamin E

Alpha-tocopherol (the body's main form of vitamin E) functions as an antioxidant, regulates cell signaling, influences immune function and inhibits coagulation. Vitamin E (tocopherols) deficiency may occur with malabsorption, cholestyramine, colestipol, isoniazid, orlistat, cystic fibrosis, celiac disease, Crohn's disease, SIBO, cirrhosis, pancreatic insufficiency, olestra, and certain anticonvulsants medications. Deficiency may result in peripheral neuropathy, ataxia, muscle weakness, retinopathy, and increased risk of CVD, prostate cancer, and cataracts. My favorite sources of vitamin E include nuts, seeds, spinach, carrots, avocado, dark leafy greens, and wheat germ. Excess vitamin E supplementation may lead to an increased propensity to bleeding issues, hemorrhagic stroke for those at risk, cramping, headaches, weakness, double vision, fatigue, diarrhea, and abdominal discomfort. Furthermore, a landmark meta-analysis showed that taking a daily dose of 400 IU or more of vitamin E was associated with an increased risk of death from all causes.[7] For this reason I recommend against routine vitamin E supplementation.

Vitamin C

Vitamin C is a powerful antioxidant involved in numerous cellular process. Some of these involve cholesterol metabolism, immune health, the synthesis of collagen, norepinephrine, and carnitine. A deficiency can result in scurvy, swollen gingiva, periodontal destruction, loose teeth, sore mouth, soft tissue ulcerations, or increased risk of infection. Increased risk of vitamin C deficiency may occur with oral contraceptives, aspirin, diuretics or NSAIDs. Excessive amounts of vitamin C can cause diarrhea, abdominal bloating, nausea, anemia, and a false positive hemoccult test. There is literature that suggests excessive use of vitamin C is a risk factor for calcium oxalate nephrolithiasis.[8] My favorite sources of vitamin C are oranges, grapefruits, strawberries, tomatos, sweet red peppers, broccoli and potatoes. I do not recommend routine vitamin C supplementation. Patients with a history of hypertension can consider 500 mg daily of vitamin C in consultation with a physician.

ALA

Alpha Lipoic Acid plays an important role in energy production, antioxidant activity, insulin signaling, cell signaling, and helps fight free radicals. Optimal levels of alpha lipoic acid may improve glucose utilization and protect against diabetic neuropathy, vascular disease, and age-related cognitive decline. ALA is found in every cell of the human body and is extremely safe at recommended doses. There are no reports of overdose but diabetics should monitor blood sugars carefully to avoid hypoglycemia. My recommended sources include spinach, broccoli, tomatoes, peas, Brussels sprouts. There is strong evidence it helps to treat the symptoms of diabetic neuropathy.[9] There are studies showing it decreases general oxidation and blood sugar.[10] I recommend diabetics consider alpha lipoic acid in a dose of 300 mg daily in consultation with a physician.

CoQ10

Coenzyme Q10 is a ubiquitous antioxidant found in every cell in the human body. It is necessary for energy production in the mitochondria. This compound helps reduce oxidative stress, improves endothelial function, decreases fatigue, improves blood flow, and lowers blood sugar and blood pressure.[11] Any patient with a history of chronic fatigue syndrome, metabolic syndrome, migraine headaches, hypertension, heart disease, on a statin, or wanting to decrease oxidation should consider taking this supplement. The healthiest sources of CoQ10 are peanuts, sesame seeds, pistachios, broccoli, cauliflower, oranges, strawberries, and legumes. I recommend patients with diabetes and hypertension take 120 mg of CoQ10 once daily with food in consultation with a physician. Also, patients with a history of migraine headaches can consider taking 100 mg of CoQ10 three times per day in consultation with a physician.

Vitamin B1

Vitamin B1 (thiamine) is necessary for production of energy, amino acids, and carbohydrates. Low levels of vitamin B1 results from use of pharmaceuticals such as diuretics, digoxin, birth control pills, or large amounts of tea and coffee. A deficiency of vitamin B1 can lead to nerve damage, dementia, heart failure, and brain damage. There is no known excessive vitamin B1 intake and no cases of overdose since the kidneys rapidly excrete excessive amounts. It is considered safe and nontoxic. My favorite sources of vitamin B1 are legumes, rice, cereal, lentils, whole grains, Brazil nuts, peas, blackstrap molasses, and spinach. I do not recommend routine vitamin B1 supplementation.

Vitamin B2

Vitamin B2 (riboflavin) is a key component in energy production, detoxification, methionine metabolism, vitamin activation, and helps fight free radicals. Risk factors for low vitamin B2 are chronic alcoholism, birth control pills, several psychiatric medications, and phenobarbital. A deficiency of riboflavin can manifest as anemia, dermatitis, stomatitis, glossitis, migraine headaches and pharyngitis. Toxicity of this vitamin is usually not seen since it is water soluable and the body doesn't absorb excessive amounts. My favorite sources of riboflavin are green vegetables, whole grains, broccoli, asparagus, spinach, mushrooms, and almonds. I do not recommend routine vitamin B2 supplementation. Patients with a history of migraine headaches can consider taking 400 mg of riboflavin daily in consultation with a physician.

Vitamin B3

Vitamin B3 (niacin) is used in energy production from food, synthesis of fatty acid, steroids, cholesterol, protein synthesis, cell signaling, and DNA repair. Niacin deficiency is uncommon in industrialized countries but is still seen in alcoholics, after bariatric surgery, or in individuals with eating disorders. Low vitamin B3 can still be seen in those individuals taking pharmaceutical drugs such as isoniazid and birth control pills. Niacin deficiency is known as pellagra and manifest as diarrhea, dementia, delusions, anxiety, insomnia, encephalopathy and dermatitis. Some well-known symptons of toxicity of niacin include elevation in liver function test, hives, flushing, nausea, vomiting, and gout attacks. Niacin has well-established antihyperlipidemic effects but because of its side effects I do not recommend it. The literature shows it increases blood sugar, increases homocysteine, and does not change clinical outcomes. My favorite sources of plant-derived B3 are whole grains, peanuts, seeds, lentils, and lima beans. I do not recommend routine vitamin B3 supplementation.

Vitamin B5

Vitamin B5 (pantothenic acid) is necessary for the formation of other fat-soluble vitamins, lipids, steroid hormones, and protein. A deficiency of B5 can manifest as nerve pain, dermatitis, and anemia. Deficiency is rare in humans and can be seen in starvation. Food sources of B5 include shitake mushrooms, avocado, sunflower seeds and sweet potatoes. As a water-soluble vitamin that can be excreted by the kidney there is no known toxicity in humans. I do not recommend routine vitamin B5 supplementation.

Vitamin B6

Vitamin B6 (pyridoxine) is used by the body to make blood sugar, neurotransmitters, red blood cells, and immune health. Deficiency in vitamin B6 is rare but risk factors include birth control pills, alcoholism, tuberculosis medication, and diuretic use. Vitamin B6 deficiency can manifest as confusion, depression, seizure, impaired immunity, increased homocysteine, irritability, dermatitis, inflamed lips and tongue. Toxicity of vitamin B6 is reported with doses above 250 mg per day and is a major concern. Some symptoms of toxicity include peripheral nerve pain, dermatitis, photosensitivity, migraine headaches, fatigue, gait abnormality, dizziness, increased liver function, and nausea. I have had several patients in my practice taking megadoses of this vitamin and they did experience some of the adverse side effects listed above. My recommendation is to get B6 from plant sources such as whole grains, vegetables, nuts, soybeans, lentils, seeds, potato, spinach, and carrots. I do not recommend routine vitamin B6 supplementation.

Vitamin B7

Vitamin B7 (biotin) is essential for synthesis of protein, DNA, carbohydrates, fatty acid, and helps the nervous system. A deficiency is rare. Symptoms of deficiency include dermatitis, fatigue, nausea, hair loss, depression, and impaired immunity. There are no known toxic effects of excess biotin consumption. My favorite sources are from whole grains, nuts, seeds, avocado, raspberries, sweet potatoes, and cauliflower. I do not recommend routine vitamin B7 supplementation.

Vitamin B9

Vitamin B9 (folic acid) is necessary for protein synthesis, the nervous system, red blood cells, and conversion of carbohydrates to energy. Folic acid is the synthetic form of B9 whereas folate is the natural form found in foods. Individuals at high risk of folate deficiency include alcoholics, those with celiac disease or inflammatory bowel disease, and those on long-term medications such as diuretics, anticonvulsants, methotrexate, and acid blockers. A deficiency can result in anemia, fatigue, increased risk of heart disease and stroke, shortness of breath, diarrhea, irritability, poor immunity, increased homocysteine, and increased risk of cancer. Excessive amounts of folic acid causing toxicity is rare. However, since folic acid is synthetic, mega doses are associated with stomach distress, nausea, anorexia, dermatitis, and seizure. Emerging literature suggests that long-term folic acid intake can increase the risk of cancer. Also, taking excessive folic acid can mask the symptoms of B12 deficiency. My favorite sources of folate are grains, green vegetables, beans, and legumes. The U.S. Preventive Task Force recommends that pregnant or breastfeeding women take 400 to 800 mcg of folic acid daily to help prevent birth defects. I recommend that most individuals get folate from whole foods such as grains, green vegetables, beans and legumes and avoid synthetic folic acid, unless you are pregnant or breastfeeding.

Vitamin B12

Vitamin B12 (cobalamin) is necessary for production of energy, synthesis of red blood cells, and nerve health. An individual may develop B12 deficiency from poor dietary intake, alcoholism, malabsorption, lack of stomach acid production, diabetic meds, and acid blocking medication. A deficiency of B12 leads to a classic constellation of symptoms. At first it may present with subtle nonspecific symptoms such as fatigue and mental fogginess. Then it can progress to more dramatic symptoms such as dementia, memory loss, nerve damage, gait abnormality, and depression. Vitamin B12 is only found in animal foods. Since the consumption of animals food is associated with heart disease, diabetes, hypertension, obesity, and cancer

I do not recommend their consumption. I recommend everyone on a plant-based diet consume 500 mcg of vitamin B12 daily.

Magnesium

Magnesium is involved in more than 300 chemical reactions in the body and important for nerve, bone, and muscle function. There is a significant association between higher intakes of magnesium and a reduced risk of diabetes.[12] Magnesium improves insulin sensitivity. Risk factors for magnesium deficiency include alcoholism, renal disease, diabetes, diuretic use, malabsorption, and parathyroid disease. Low magnesium may manifest as weakness, spasms, depression, hypertension, arrhythmias, and personality changes. Excessive magnesium may manifest as low blood pressure, nausea, vomiting, diarrhea, weakness, facial flushing, and irregular heart beat. I recommend getting magnesium from foods such as green leafy vegetables, legumes, nuts, seeds, soybeans, oatmeal, buckwheat, avocados, and brown rice. Diabetics should consider taking 400 mg of magnesium glycinate daily with food, in consultation with a physician to help monitor blood sugars. I do not recommend routine magnesium supplementation.

Zinc

Zinc is a cofactor for more than 300 enzymes and is needed for cell growth, reproduction, immune function, vision, wound healing, and collagen. Zinc is a mineral that has shown promising effects in lower blood sugar and is a powerful antioxidant. Zinc supplementation in patients with diabetes showed beneficial effects on blood sugar control and lipids. Zinc deficiency can manifest with hair loss, skin rash, impaired immunity, impaired sexual function, and altered taste and smell. Excessive zinc can manifest as nausea, vomiting, diarrhea, abdominal pain, dizziness, irritability, headache, and lethargy. Risk factors for deficiency are malabsorption, excessive alcohol, chronic diarrhea, and chronic diuretic use. Diabetics can consider a dosage of zinc 15 to 30 mg per day depending on your diet and in conjunction with your physician. I do not recommend routine zinc supplementation.

Essential Fatty Acids

Omega-3 fatty acids are essential nutrients that cannot be synthesized by the human body. They must be obtained from dietary sources. The Standard American Diet is largely deficient in healthy omega-3s. A deficiency is associated with dry skin, dermatitis, poor wound healing, increased risk of infection, increased cardiovascular disease and increased inflammation. Excessive omega-3 supplementation can lead to an impaired immune system and increased cholesterol. There is an association between higher alpha-linolenic acid (short chain omega-3 fatty acid) and moderately lower risk of cardiovascular disease.[13] We know that C-reactive protein (CRP) is a marker of systemic inflammation and is linked to heart disease. A diet rich in alpha-linolenic acid can help decrease inflammation and decrease the risk of cardiovascular disease.[14] My favorite dietary sources of omega-3s include flax-seeds, chia seeds, walnuts, soybeans, cauliflower, tofu, and fresh herbs. Long-chain fatty acids DHA/EPA, such the ones found in fish and algae, offer numerous health benefits. Dietary short-chain fatty acid alpha-linolenic acid (ALA) can be converted to DHA/EPA but conversion is limited to 0 to 8 percent. Thus, it is important to consume DHA/EPA regularly and not rely on endogenous conversion. DHA/EPA can help decrease triglycerides, blood pressure, endothelial dysfunction, and thrombosis while increasing myocardial efficiency.[15] In short, regular consumption of EPA/DHA in one's diet can help with cardiovascular health by preventing progression of atherosclerosis, decreasing the risks of coronary restenosis, myocardial infarction, and sudden cardiac death.[16-18] I have concerns about regular consumption of fish because of the potential risk of methylmercury, dioxins, polychlorinated biphenyls, polybrominated diphenyl ethers, and pesticides. Although commercially available fish oils remove these pollutants, I do not recommend fish oil because of the long-term sustainability and the negative environmental impact. I recommend 250 mg of micro-algae derived DHA/EPA daily for anyone on a plant-based diet to get adequate long chain fatty acid. I recommend taking 1-2 tablespoons of organic ground flax seeds for short-chain fatty acid alpha-linolenic acid (ALA). Avoid refined oils.

Turmeric

Turmeric is a spice found in curry and is commonly used in Ayurvedic cooking. This spice also plays a central role in the diet of Okinawan elders, one of the longest lived cultures in the world. The active compound in turmeric is curcumin, which has anti-inflammatory and anti-cancer properties. Curcumin also decreases oxidation, pain and inflammation, and C-reactive protein.[19] On the days that I do not eat curry, I take turmeric capsules with 1,000 mg of curcumin. Use capsules that contain black pepper (piperine) to enhance absorption.

Pearls from Chapter 9

Ideally, one would get all the essential vitamins, minerals, and phytochemicals from the foods that we eat. As Hippocrates noted several millennia ago, food is medicine. A whole-food, low glycemic, plant-based diet will give all the micronutrients necessary for health. For most, a whole-food based multivitamin, vitamin D, vitamin B12, alpha-linolenic acid (ALA), and a DHA/EPA supplement are important in order to avoid any nutritional deficiency. This is a safety net, not a substitute for a healthy diet!

Chapter 9 Endnotes

1. Guallar E, Stranges S, Mulrow C, Appel LJ, Miller ER. Enough Is Enough: Stop Wasting Money on Vitamin and Mineral Supplements. *Ann Intern Med.* 2013;159(12):850-851. doi:107326/0003-4819-159-12-201312170-00011.

2. Anton S, Leeuwenburgh C. Fasting or caloric restriction for Healthy Aging. *Exp Gerontol.* 2013;48(10):1003-1005. doi:101016/jexger201304011.

3. Erridge C, Attina T, Spickett CM, Webb DJ. A high-fat meal induces low-grade endotoxemia: evidence of a novel mechanism of postprandial inflammation. *Am J Clin Nutr.* 2007;86(5):1286-1292.

4. The effect of vitamin E and beta carotene on the incidence of lung cancer and other cancers in male smokers. The Alpha-Tocopherol, Beta Carotene Cancer Prevention Study Group. *N Engl J Med.* 1994;330(15):1029-1035.

5. Omenn GS, Goodman GE, Thornquist M.D., et al. Effects of a combination of beta carotene and vitamin A on lung cancer and cardiovascular disease. *N Engl J Med.* 1996;334(18):1150-1155.

6. Vivekananthan DP, Penn MS, Sapp SK, Hsu A, Topol EJ. Use of antioxidant vitamins for the prevention of car-diovascular disease: meta-analysis of randomised trials. *Lancet.* 2003;361(9374):2017-2023.

7. Miller ER, Pastor-Barriuso R, Dalal D, Riemersma RA, Appel LJ, Guallar E. Meta-Analysis: High-Dosage Vita-min E Supplementation May Increase All-Cause Mortal-ity. *Ann Intern Med.* 2005;142(1):37-46. doi:107326/0003-4819-142-1-200501040-00110.

8. Massey LK, Liebman M, Kynast-Gales SA. Ascorbate

increases human oxaluria and kidney stone risk. *J Nutr.* 2005;135(7):1673-1677.

9. Golbidi S, Badran M, Laher I. Diabetes and Alpha Lipoic Acid. *Front Pharmacol.* 2011;2:69 doi:103389/ fphar201100069.

10. Gomes MB, Negrato CA. Alpha-lipoic acid as a pleiotropic compound with potential therapeutic use in diabetes and other chronic diseases. *Diabetol Metab Syndr.* 2014;6(1):80. doi:101186/1758-5996-6-80.

11. Hodgson JM, Watts GF, Playford DA, Burke V, Croft KD. Coenzyme Q10 improves blood pressure and glycaemic control: a controlled trial in subjects with type 2 diabetes. *Eur J Clin Nutr.* 2002;56(11):1137-1142.

12. Dong JY, Xun P, He K, Qin LQ. Magnesium Intake and Risk of Type 2 Diabetes: Meta-analysis of prospective cohort studies *Diabetes Care.* 2011;34(9):2116-2122. doi:102337/dc11-0518.

13. Pan A, Chen M, Chowdhury R, et al. α-Linolenic acid and risk of cardiovascular disease: a systematic review and meta-analysis. *Am J of Clin Nutr.* 2012;96(6):1262-1273. doi:103945/ajcn112044040.

14. Zhao G, Etherton TD, Martin KR, West SG, Gillies PJ, Kris-Etherton PM. Dietary alpha-linolenic acid reduces inflammatory and lipid cardiovascular risk factors in hypercholesterolemic men and women. *J Nutr.* 2004;134(11):2991-2997.

15. Mozaffarian D, Wu JH. Omega-3 fatty acids and cardiovascular disease: effects on risk factors, molecular pathways, and clinical events. *J Am Coll Cardiol.* 2011;58(20):2047-2067. doi: 101016/jjacc201106063.

16. Mozaffarian D, Lemaitre RN, King IB, et al. Plasma Phospholipid Long-Chain Omega-3 Fatty Acids and Total and Cause-Specific Mortality in Older Adults: the Cardiovascular Health Study. *Ann Intern Med.* 2013;158(7):515-525. doi:107326/0003-4819-158-7-201304020-00003.

17. Mozaffarian D, Wu Jason. Fatty Acids and Cardiovascular Health: Are Effects of EPA and DHA Shared or Complementary? *J Nutr.* 2012;142(3):S614-625.

18. Kromhout D. Omega-3 fatty acids and coronary heart disease. The final verdict? *Curr Opin Lipidol.* 2012 Dec;23(6):554-559. doi: 101097/MOL0b013e328359515f.

19. Jurenka JS. Anti-inflammatory properties of curcumin, a major constituent of Curcuma longa: a review of preclinical and clinical research. *Altern Med Rev.* 2009;14(2):141-153.

Part Three

Movement in
Moderation is Your
Fountain of Youth

CHAPTER TEN

THE FOUNTAIN OF YOUTH: EXERCISE

Physical fitness is not only one of the most important keys to a healthy body, it is the basis of dynamic and creative intellectual activity.

—JOHN F. KENNEDY

If we could give every individual the right amount of nourishment and exercise, not too little and not too much, we would have found the safest way to health.

—HIPPOCRATES

A PATIENT OF MINE IS A HEALTHY, VIVACIOUS NONA-genarian in her late nineties. She has a lucid memory, is at her ideal body weight, and is in perfect health. One of her secrets to exceptional longevity is daily exercise for more than eighty years. Her baseline physical activity involves gardening and walking, however she also makes time for health-promoting physical activity.

Human beings have evolved to be bipedal and spend the majority of our waking hours standing. The human body was designed to move, walk, stand, run, etc. The only stationary eight hours of your day should be when you are lying horizontal while sleeping. Sitting is a disease. There is an accumulating body of research that shows your time spent sitting is an independent risk factor for mortality or premature death independent of your exercise. In other words, if you exercise intensely, biking, swimming, or running for one hour per day but then spend the rest of your day sitting, you are at risk for premature death. It is that simple. James Levine, M.D., Ph.D., Professor of Medicine at Mayo Clinic Arizona, states that "Human beings evolved as walking entities, exploring the world on our feet." Furthermore, sitting, in and of itself, causes harm to your body. Dr. Levine goes on to state: "The strangest thing in the world is that people spend all day scrunched in a chair. It's a form of physical entrapment."

What happens to your body when you sit? Research shows that sitting leads to lowered metabolic rate, muscle atrophy, increased LDL, decreased insulin sensitivity, bone loss, cognitive decline, arterial damage, increased risk of type 2 diabetes, weight gain, and premature death.[1] To most folks, this does not come as a surprise. If you sit too much, you are being sedentary and being sedentary leads to disease. This is intuitive. Cardiologist David Alter, M.D., states: "Avoiding sedentary time and getting regular exercise are both important for improving your health and survival." Dr. Alter published an analysis of forty-seven articles that found the amount of time a person sits during the day is associated with a 15 to 20 percent risk of death from any cause, 15 to 20 percent higher risk of heart disease and death from heart disease, 15 to 20 percent higher risk of cancer and death from cancer, and a 90 percent higher risk of diabetes, regardless of regular exercise.[2]

The study found that current guidelines recommend that most people should engage in at least 250 minutes per week of moderate vigorous physical activity to help one lose weight. This amount of exercise will also help prevent many chronic diseases especially heart disease, diabetes, obesity and several types of cancers. However, 150 minutes of exercise per week is adequate to maintain weight and still confers all the listed health benefits listed, if you are at your ideal body weight. These recommendations come from the American College of Sports Medicine, in an attempt to help with the obesity crisis in America. These recommendations are in line with the Physical Activity Guidelines for Americans released by the government in 2008. However, they go one step further. Since exercise has such powerful benefits, they recommend 300 minutes per week of aerobic exercise (five hours).

Exercise is the fountain of youth. Regular aerobic exercise is an excellent strategy to help prevent chronic disease and extend the human lifespan. Research studies show an association between regular exercise and lowering the risk of premature death, heart disease, stroke, high blood pressure, metabolic syndrome, type 2 diabetes, colon cancer, breast cancer, lung cancer, endometrial cancer, and depression. Exercise increases bone density, sleep quality, muscle mass, cognitive function, cardiopulmonary fitness, well-being, and functional health in older adults. Exercise also decreases LDL cholesterol and triglycerides while improving HDL cholesterol, endothelial function, and insulin sensitivity. Exercise reduces abdominal obesity, helps prevent falls, and helps with weight loss and weight maintenance after weight loss. With aging, we start losing bone strength, muscle mass, and suffer damage and senescence to a trillion cells in our bodies. With exercise, we promote healthy aging by releasing vascular endothelial growth factor to keep arteries healthy, we promote brain-derived neurotrophic factor to help keep our brains healthy, and we promote the production of mitochondria in cells to help energy production. In effect, when you exercise you are promoting a healthy heart, brain, bones, muscles, and metabolism and in essence delaying and reversing the effects of aging.

The World Health Organization recommends 150 minutes of aerobic exercise per week for optimal health. It is important to remember that any exercise is better than none. We know that even thirty minutes per week will offer benefits.

A meta-analysis study published in *JAMA* in 2009 studied 102,980 participants and found that the all-cause mortality was related to cardiorespiratory fitness.[3] The lower the fitness level the higher the risk of all-cause mortality. In this study, participants with a maximal exercise capacity of 7.9 METS (Metabolic Equivalent of Task) or higher had a lower risk of death from any cause. Anything above 6 METS is considered vigorous physical activity, such as jogging. Sexual activity almost made cut, as it came in at a close 5.8 METS. I give a practical recommendation of exercise every day (vigorous walking is great) for at least one hour. Getting individuals who are sedentary to move will automatically increase physical fitness. Movement helps prevent premature death.

There is a significant inverse relationship between vigorous activity and mortality.[4] This study linked exercise and all-cause mortality. It sampled 204,542 adults ages forty-five to seventy-five years from Australia. Among those reporting any moderate to vigorous activity, those who had vigorous activity had a lower all-cause mortality.

The negative effects of a sedentary lifestyle are similar to the negative health effects of being in outer space. Being in outer space for an extended period of time leads to dramatic changes in human physiology including bone loss or osteoporosis, muscle atrophy and sarcopenia, decompensation of fitness and decreased cardiovascular health. To combat these negative health effects, astronauts tie themselves down to a treadmill to get exercise while in outer space. We don't need to undertake such drastic measures here on earth as gravity is our friend. One of the most crucial things you can do for your health is avoid prolonged sitting. For starters, I would avoid sitting for more than four hours a day and ideally you can spend most of your work day standing. Standing desks have become very popular and, surprisingly, a lot of employers are recommending them. Furthermore, I would recommend a daily one-hour walk at the very minimum. Studies from across the world have shown that exceptional longevity is associated with physical activity.

Pearls from Chapter 10

Exercise is the fountain of youth. Regular aerobic exercise is an excellent strategy to help prevent chronic disease and extend the human lifespan. Research studies show an association between regular exercise and lowering the risk of premature death, heart disease, stroke, high blood pressure, metabolic syndrome, type 2 diabetes, colon cancer, breast cancer, lung cancer, endometrial cancer, and depression. Exercise increases bone density, sleep quality, muscle mass, cognitive function, cardiopulmonary fitness, well-being, and functional health in older adults. Exercise also improves HDL cholesterol, decreases LDL cholesterol, decrease triglycerides, improves endothelial function, improves insulin sensitivity. Exercise reduces abdominal obesity, helps prevent falls, and helps with weight loss and weight maintenance. I recommend one hour a day of physical activity and this could be as simple as vigorous walking. Also, I recommend that everyone avoid prolonged sitting. Sitting has negative consequences on human health independent of how much exercise.

Chapter 10 Endnotes

1. Wilmot EG, Edwardson CL, Achana FA, et al. Sedentary time in adults and the association with diabetes, cardiovascular disease and death: systematic review and meta-analysis. *Diabetologia.* 2012;55(11):2895-2905. doi: 101007/s00125-012-2677-z.

2. Biswas A, Oh PI, Faulkner GE, et al. Sedentary time and its association with risk for disease incidence, mortality, and hospitalization in adults: a systematic review and meta-analysis. *Ann Intern Med.* 2015;162(2):123-132. doi: 107326/M14-1651.

3. Kodama S1, Saito K, Tanaka S, et al. Cardiorespiratory fitness as a quantitative predictor of all-cause mortality and cardiovascular events in healthy men and women: a meta-analysis. *JAMA.* 2009;301(19):2024-2035. doi: 101001/jama2009681.

4. Gebel K, Ding D, Chey T, Stamatakis E, Brown WJ, Bauman AE. Effect of Moderate to Vigorous Physical Activity on All-Cause Mortality in Middle-aged and Older Australians. *JAMA Intern Med.* 2015;175(6):970-977. doi: 101001/jamainternmed20150541.

CHAPTER ELEVEN

PRACTICAL STEPS FOR EXERCISING

Do what you can, with what you have, where you are.
—THEODORE ROOSEVELT

Exercise is amazing, from the inside out. I feel so alive and have more energy.
—VANESSA HUDGENS

THE HEALTHIEST FORM OF EXERCISE IS THE ONE that you actually perform versus being sedentary. In other words, any form of exercise is healthier than not exercising. From research studies around the world we know that exceptional longevity is associated with movement. To reap the health benefits of exercise one does not have to invest in expensive equipment, gym membership, CrossFit, P90X, or do excessive strenuous sports such as ultramarathons, Ironman triathlons, or marathons. In fact, the best form of exercise is walking all day and avoiding sitting. There is exercise built in to the everyday activities of the longest lived cultures. So how do you start an exercise program?

Initially, it is important to define one's current activity level. Baseline activity level is essentially the activity that one performs in their day-to-day life, for example, doing housework, walking the dog, and going up and down steps. The baseline activity level of people in most industrialized countries is considerably lower than in Third World countries. We drive to work and the grocery store instead of walking or biking. Many of us are employed in desk jobs, and we purchase packaged foods. Our lives contrast with cultures such as Okinawa, Japan and Sardinia, Italy which are known for exceptionally longevity.[1] Those citizens remain physically active throughout the day in the field or working in garden, and walking is their main source of transportation. A healthy level of physical activity is part of every-day living and in these cultures they don't need extra physical activity beyond baseline. However, in America, usually, our baseline activity level is not enough for optimal health. In sedentary cultures like in America, there is a need for what is defined as health-enhancing physical activity.[2] Some examples of health-enhancing physical activity include vigor-ous walking, dancing, swimming, yoga, mowing the lawn, bicycling, hiking, jogging, and weight training, etc. Check with your doctor before embarking on any health-enhancing physical activity beyond your baseline activity level.

Exercise can be classified in three broad cat-egories that are interrelational. The three types are aerobic, resistance, and flexibility. If you enhance one, you automatically improve the other. Aerobic exercise, also known as "cardio," involves activities such as a vigorous walking, swimming, cycling, jogging, hiking, etc. that you can perform for up to an hour or two. These actions primarily work on cardiopulmonary fitness. Resistance or anaerobic training generally involves weights or another form of high-intensity exercise where the body enters significant oxygen debt. This form of exercise is designed to promote strength, speed, and power. Some examples include interval workouts, sprinting, jump rope, vigorous hiking, and weight training. These activities lead to oxygen debt and anaerobic metabolism in as little as two minutes.

Flexibility is the range of motion in muscle or joints. It allows one to perform day-to-day activities such as squatting, bending, rising up from bed, getting into a car seat, etc. Flexibility keeps the body limber and healthy and prevents injury. It may also improve athletic performance. There are four types of stretches: static, dynamic, passive and active. Yoga is my favorite form of flexibility training since it incorporates all four types of stretches.

The optimum exercise I recommend is any one that you perform. Health-promoting physical activity should become a habit. Once daily exercise has become a habit, this will engender long-term success with your health plan. I learned a mnemonic device from one of my mentors at Mayo Clinic: DIDKISMIF 30. This mnemonic device will help you remember that when you pick a physical activity make it practical. DIDKISMIF 30 stands for: Do it Daily, Keep it Simple, Make it Fun, for thirty minutes today. In other words, if you choose your physical activity to be swimming, but you do not have a swimming pool in the backyard and you cannot invest $10,000 to build one and your nearest swimming pool is three hours away, I suggest that swimming NOT be your exercise of choice to get in shape. If you love to dance and there are many dance clubs in your local community then using dancing as a form of physical fitness to get you healthy is an outstanding choice. Maybe you will choose something you can do easily in your house with or without a partner. Make it something you can do daily. It should be simple and fun. Then you will more likely be able to maintain this activity for a long time and you will reap the benefits.

A sample week of exercise can be a moderate walk four days per week and a yoga class three times per week. This plan gives one a good blend of aerobic, anaerobic, and flexibility training for the week. Those who cannot go to a yoga class can do the following plan. Walk for one hour on four days per week and perform a routine of lunges, push ups, jump rope, dips, pull ups, and sit ups on the remaining three days per week.

One fitness tool I highly recommend is a heart rate monitor so you can monitor your fitness level and ensure adequate effort. When using a heart rate monitor you should first calculate your maximum heart rate. A simple guideline for someone who is less than forty years old is to take 220 minus your age and the difference is your maximum heart rate. A more sophisticated calculation is to take your age, multiply it by 0.7 and subtract the product from 208.[3] As an example, I am thirty-nine years old, so from the simplistic calculation of 220 minus my age my maximum heart rate is 181. From the more sophisticated method I use my age thirty-nine times 0.7 which equals 180.7. In my case both numbers are fairly accurate since my current max heart rate as measured during an road race is 185. Once you have found your maximum heart rate then use your heart rate monitor as a training tool.

For maximum benefit, exercise so that your heart rate is 60 to 80 percent of maximum for thirty to sixty minutes. When planning an aerobic work-out, allow additional time for the warm up (getting to recommended heart rate) and a cool down (gradually allowing your heart rate to come down). Here is a sample calculation: my maximum heart rate is 185 x .60 and 185 x .80 and this equals 111 to 148. I want to maintain my heart rate in the range of 111 to 148 for thirty to sixty minutes, four days each week.

At least two or sometimes three times per week, I recommend getting ten to twenty minutes of anaerobic exercise, defined as heart rate at 80 to 100 percent of maximum. On the two or three times per week that I perform anaerobic exercise, my heart rate is between 148 and 185. Since you are in oxygen debt, this form of exercise should be performed in intervals from several seconds to no more than several minutes. Since anaerobic training is more intense, the body needs more time to recover so I recommend at least one recovery day between this type of workout. A good guideline, for those who don't have a heart rate monitor to measure the intensity level of a workout, is to use your breathing as a guide. If you can carry on a conversation speaking in full sentences, you are likely in the aerobic zone. If you are having difficulty carrying on a conversation and speaking in short sentences, or just using one-word responses, you are likely in the anaerobic zone.

In summary, the healthiest form of exercise is the one that you actually perform versus being sedentary. From research studies around the world we know that exceptional longevity is associated with movement. The key is to pick a simple and fun exercise plan and stick to it daily. Since the three forms of exercise are interrelational, if you improve one you automatically improve the other, like a holographic body. I recommend thirty minutes of moderate physical activity on most days of the week.[4]

Pearls from Chapter 11

When choosing an exercise plan remember the following practical advice: Keep it simple, Do it Daily, and Make it Fun for 30 minutes each day. Each week incorporate a good balance of aerobic, anaerobic, and flexibility training for optimum fitness. With exercise, you promote healthy aging by releasing vascular endothelial growth factor to keep your arteries healthy, brain-derived neurotrophic factor to help keep your brain healthy, and the production of mitochondria in cells to help energy production. In effect, when you exercise, you are promoting a healthy heart, brain, bones, muscles and metabolism, and, in essence, you are delaying and reversing the effects of aging.

Chapter 11 Endnotes

1. Buettner D. *The Blue Zones: Lessons for Living Longer From the People Who've Lived the Longest.* 2nd ed. Washington, DC: National Geographic; 2012.

2. Physical Activity Guidelines. Office of Disease Prevention and Health Promotion website. http://health.gov/paguidelines/guidelines/chapter1.aspx.

3. Tanaka H, Monahan KD, Seals DR. Age-predicted maximal heart rate revisited. *J Am Coll Cardiol.* 2001;37(1):153-156.

4. Physical Activity and Health: A Report of the Surgeon General. Centers for Disease Control and Prevention website. http://www.cdc.gov/nccdphp/sgr/summ.htm.

CHAPTER TWELVE

DANGERS OF EXERCISE

Balance is good, because one extreme or the other leads to misery, and I've spent a lot of my life at one of those extremes.

—TRENT REZNOR

If one oversteps the bounds of moderation, the greatest pleasures cease to please.

—EPICTETUS

A FORTY-FIVE-YEAR-OLD PATIENT OF MINE WENT from couch to training for his first marathon. He presented to my clinic with profound fatigue, decreased libido, and increased body fat even though he was exercising more frequently and more intensely. He also suffered a stress fracture. He was diagnosed with hypogonadism from overtraining syndrome. An appropriate adjustment to his training schedule that allowed for adequate rest provided healing for a full recovery.

Exercise is the Fountain of Youth as discussed in the previous chapter. However, as illustrated in the case, exercise is not without its dangers. We have all heard of professional and elite runners who have died of sudden cardiac death during a marathon. Does this mean people should not run marathons? No. In fact, you have a higher risk of dying driving your car to the starting line of a marathon than you do of dying while running a marathon.[1] Sudden cardiac death during a marathon is an extremely rare event, with only one death per 100,000 participants. Whereas dying in a motor vehicle collision is approximately ten deaths per 100,000 drivers. So driving a car is ten times riskier than a marathon. The health benefits of training for a marathon as discussed in previous chapters are overwhelming in the support of exercising.

There are dangers of exercising. Those dangers include musculoskeletal injury, sudden cardiac death, myocardial infarction, rhabdomyolysis, bronchoconstriction, hyperthermia, amenorrhea and infertility, and hyponatremia. Some of these dangers are easily avoided by training appropriately, hydration, and some simple safety measures.

However, the more concerning issue with exercise is whether too much exercise is dangerous to the heart muscle. A recent article in the *Mayo Clinic Proceedings* suggests there is a threshold in terms of the amount of exercise that offers health benefits.[2] Beyond this threshold level, there are diminishing returns and can lead to adverse cardiovascular consequences.

Chronic intense and sustained exercise can create pathological changes in the heart muscle in endurance sports, especially marathons, ultramarathons, and triathlons. We have known for many years in the medical community that endurance athletes have a five-fold increase prevalence of atrial fibrillation. However, these new findings of pathological changes of the heart tissue with an associated elevation of biomarkers, such as binaturetic peptid (BNP) and cardiac troponin, that are seen in myocardial injury is concerning. In this article, Dr. O'Keefe and colleagues suggest that approximately one hour a day of aerobic exercise and about seventy-five minutes per week of high intensity is safe. This recommendation is in line with the major associations from American College of Sports Medicine, the Institute of Medicine, and governmental recommendations.

Even though there is emerging literature that excessive endurance exercise is harmful for the heart, the overwhelming consensus is that exercising is better for you than not exercising. Routine physical activity, such as walking an hour a day, gardening, biking, swimming, hiking, and dancing, up to an hour a day, is safe. The danger lies in excessive endurance sports, such as Ironman, ultramarathoning, marathons, century bike rides, marathon swimming, etc. This category of exercise places an overload on the cardiovascular system without appropriate rest. It has been my clinical experience that many athletes perform endurance sports to an extreme level without allowing adequate rest for the body. Literature shows that this amount of physical activity can lead to what's known as overtraining syndrome. The mechanism that leads to overtraining syndrome has still not been fully elucidated but involves disruption to the endocrine system, immune system, and affects the hypothalamic pituitary axis.[3] Over time the athlete has a decrease in athletic performance and can have a myriad of symptoms including fatigue, chronic infections, depression, weakness, irritability, agitation, tachycardia, loss of motivation, insomnia, stiff muscles, etc. There is a sports training cycle (periodization) for improving your physical fitness that involves stress, rest, recover, and repeat. The rest and recovery portion of training is actually the most important to ensure adequate recovery and optimal performance. An Olympian once told me that any fool can train hard as hell but it takes a genius to know how to recover. In other words, the key is moderation.

An individual can avoid overtraining and negative consequences with some simple time-honored methods. First and most important is to control stress. Uncontrolled stress as discussed in the first part of the book can lead to insomnia, fatigue, aging, heart disease, cancer, hypertension, excess of cortisol, diabetes, and depression. Also, the athlete must get adequate sleep for recovery after an intense training load. Furthermore, excessive racing and competition creates stress and hampers the body's ability to recover. The moral of the story is everything in moderation.

There is a parable that summarizes the path of moderation very well. The Buddha was following extreme aesthetic practices as a means to attain enlightenment or self-realization. He was on the verge of death from severe malnutrition and was cachectic from near starvation. A beautiful maiden saw him as a near corpse and fed him a bowl of rice. His brother monks paradoxically thought that this was a radical move for the Buddha to take food from a lady and felt that he had fallen from the path to enlightenment. The Buddha, after being revived and energized by food, was inspired by the following ancient song:

> *Fair goes the dancing when the Sitar is tuned.*
> *Tune us the Sitar neither high nor low,*
> *And we will dance away the hearts of men.*
> *But the string too tight breaks, and the music*
>   *dies.*
> *The string too slack has no sound, and the*
>   *music dies.*
> *There is a middle way.*
> *Tune us the Sitar neither low nor high.*
> *And we will dance away the hearts of men.*

This ancient song that inspired the Buddha has profound significance for overall health. Sitting in a lotus posture for three hours every morning will not guarantee enlightenment or make you a better person. Similarly, following a radical diet or exercise plan will lead to relapse because in the long term these health plans are not sustainable. Extreme diet and exercise plans lead to more stress. Furthermore, these unhealthy habits can be unhealthy in themselves. Moderation is a good thing and the key to longterm success. Remember the famous aphorism, "The perfect is the enemy of the good."

PEARLS FROM CHAPTER 12

The benefits of daily vigorous aerobic exercise greatly outweigh the harms of not exercising. There is a sweet spot, a goldilocks zone, of not too much and not too little exercise for optimal health and disease prevention. I would recommend daily aerobic exercise of up to one hour per day and no more than sixty to seventy-five minutes of high intensity exercise per week. There is a law of diminishing returns. More exercise than the current guidelines suggest, in terms of intensity and volume, could, over time, damage the heart muscle.

CHAPTER 12 ENDNOTES

1. Redelmeier DA, Greenwald JA. Competing risks of mortality with marathons: retrospective analysis. *BMJ*. 2007;335(7633):1275-1277. doi:101136/bmj3938455153925.

2. O'Keefe JH, Patil HR, Lavie CJ, Magalski A, Vogel RA, McCullough PA. Potential Adverse Cardiovascular Effects From Excessive Endurance Exercise. *Mayo Clin Proc*. 2012;87(6):587-595 doi:101016/jmayocp201204005.

3. Kreher JB, Schwartz JB. Overtraining Syndrome: A Practical Guide. *Sports Health*. 2012;4(2):128-138. doi:101177/1941738111434406.

LIVE YOUR DREAM

Life is a dream for the wise,
a game for the fool,
a comedy for the rich,
a tragedy for the poor.
—SHOLOM ALEICHEM

Shoot for the moon, because even if you miss, you'll land in the stars.
—LES BROWN

Be happy in the moment, that's enough. Each moment is all we need,
not more.
—MOTHER TERESA

IT IS A FACT THAT OUR HUMAN BODY IS EPHEMERAL and fleeting. In the vastness of the cosmos and the immensity of time, humans live but for a fleeting moment. Our bodies are recycled stardust and our time on earth is but a few seconds when compared to billions of years of earth's existence. Think of your body as a rental house. How are you currently taking care of your rental house? Are you treating it kindly and allowing it to be a vehicle for self-actualization, liberation, and enlightenment? You must treat your rental house with care since it is your true home. Your rental house only has one address: the present moment, the here and now.

It is a scientific fact that your body is slowly burning. Your average body temperature is 98.6 Fahrenheit, which is a slow smoldering burn. Everyone eventually must "shuffle off this mortal coil." The question is: "When will your rental house burn down to the ground, and go back to the earth from where it came?" You have a powerful thermostat to control the temperature of your rental house. You can lower the temperature by following the three steps for superior health and set the thermostat that will allow for maximum longevity and health. Or, you can commit crimes against wisdom and adjust this metaphorical thermostat, to increase the burn rate of your body, your rental house. Health and longevity is a choice. Superior health is your inheritance and how your body was designed to function.

The famous poem by Oliver Wendell Holmes about the one-hoss shay is a perfect analogy for the design of the human body (our rental house). In Holmes' poem, the one-hoss shay was built in such a logical way it stayed fully functional the entire way. It was precisely built, in a logical way, to last exactly 100 years to the day. Then Holmes states the one-hoss shay "went to pieces all at once, and nothing first, — just as bubbles do when they burst."

Similarly, the human body is designed to live 100 to 120 years with robust, vibrant, superior health. For example, the longest lived human in recorded history is Jeanne Louise Calment, who lived a vibrant and full life to the age of 122. She has set the gold standard of what humans can do. It is reported that she remained lucid until the very end. And at the end of this period, of fully active and engaged living, like the one-hoss shay, the rental body crumbles and falls apart at the end of its natural lifespan. The average American turns up the thermostat and accelerates the rate of consumption, entropy, and decay of the rental house, our precious body. Modern lifestyle causes a large scolding flame and heat that metaphorically represents disease, pain, and suffering. It leads to premature death as the human body is exhausted and burns and crumbles at fifty to seventy years of age. It is an early visitation by the Grim Reaper.

This does not have to be the case. Our natural state, our birth right, is superior health.

Superior health is your true home. Superior health comes naturally to children. Children effortlessly experience and express satchitananda. Satchitananda is a sanskrit word that means true existence, spontaneous knowledge of the truth, and pure bliss. When you look at a child expressing joy, happiness, love, creativity, inquisitiveness, spontaneity, boundless energy, and a zest for life, realize that this is your natural inheritance! Movement and exercise for a child comes easily and naturally. Children also naturally resonate with healthy foods like vegetables and fruits. Most children are free of mental stress. This is our natural state.

Part of having great health is following your heart's every desire and allowing your dreams to manifest. Children, with their zest and joy for life, are dreamers. This is a good thing, and healthy. Adults dream at night but never dream big with their eyes open during waking hours. The zestfull joy of big dreams has vanished and is gone forever. Why do adults lose this amazing capacity to dream with open eyes? Chronic uncontrolled stress is what zaps the zest for life!

Pain and hardships are universal: they exist in human life, regardless of your station. However, mental stress, worrying, and anxiety over events that one cannot control creates suffering. This type of mental worrying that creates suffering is unnecessary. Through meditation and mindfulness we reduce and control stress and avoid unnecessary suffering. Once we reduce stress we can experience satchitananda and pursue our dreams.

Having a dream to shoot for on a day-to-day basis creates the journey. If you have struggled with stress, weight gain, and chronic disease, then make a commitment to achieve superior health. Have the dream that you will prevent and even reverse chronic disease! By controlling stress through mindfulness and meditation, nutritional excellence, and appropriate exercise, your dream will become a reality.

On this journey to superior health there will be challenges. It is important to keep mindfulness of the present moment also known as witness consciousness. Keep in mind the interrelationship of thoughts, emotions, and behavior. Negative thoughts and emotions will rise up from a dark place, perhaps on a daily basis. However, you have the power to control your behavior. Realize those thoughts and emotions are not the real you. Thoughts and emotions will come and go without your conscious control. The key is to develop mindfulness and consciously become aware of your every action. By consciously becoming aware of your behavior, you control your destiny. You will choose behaviors that are health-promoting. There is a wonderful quote by T. Harv Eker that drives this point home: "How you do anything is how you do everything." When one trains the mind to be present with the simple things in life, then when big stressors arise one can be fully present and choose a healthy response.

There is a powerful story of one of my personal heros, Mahatma Gandhi, who achieved superior health, and knew how to dream big with his eyes open. It is said that a Western journalist once asked him, "Mr. Gandhi, you've been working fifteen hours a day for fifty years. Don't you ever feel like taking a few weeks off and going for a vacation?" Gandhi laughed and said, "Why? I am always on vacation."[1] That is the secret. Every action should bring joy and freedom. One of Gandhi's favorite books, the Bhagavad Gita, summarizes this principle well and shows why Gandhi was always fulfilled: "Let your concern be with action alone and never with the fruits of action. Do not let the results of action be your motive … perform your actions renouncing attachments, indifferent to success and failure."

As children we always dream big and do not think consciously of the mechanics of our dreams' fulfillment. This is a wonderful thing. We have colorful dreams at night but also have many vivid dreams during waking hours. We have infinite potential as children. We dream of being astronauts, soccer players, movie stars, and super heroes. As adults, we become calloused by the monotony of day-to-day reality. We lose our capacity to dream big and when this happens we lose vitality and zest for life. Also, this leads to aging. As George Bernard Shaw said, "We don't stop playing because we grow old, we grow old because we stop playing."

Chasing your dreams and keeping them alive should happen effortlessly and in many ways synchronistically. Dreams are a great way to keep a zest for life and serve as guideposts to achieve grand and wondrous things. It is said that a conspiracy of improbable events come together and bring about something unusual, unexpected, and miraculous. The key is to make a commitment to follow the three steps: plan your week, try your best every day, and let go of the results. If you try your best every day, nothing more and nothing less, you will reap the benefits of the plan in the short-term and the long-term.

As you embark on the three steps for superior health, remember this fact. The product, end results, and fruits of one's labor are not the most important things. The number on the scale is not the most important thing. The most fulfilling and important thing is the process, the journey, the road, the labor one puts in while aiming for the goal. Most adults lose this powerful, present-moment awareness. Research shows that the default mode of humans is of mind-wandering, which correlates with unhappiness. One excellent way to combat this natural tendency of mind-wandering is through meditation.[2] Through meditation we can activate the brain regions to help ourselves focus on the present moment and increase happiness. This will also allow us to focus on the task at hand. Our dreams and goals manifest spontaneously as a by-product.

Your health destiny is superior health. Your true home is a state of superior health where you experience true existence, spontaneous knowing of the truth, and bliss of being alive. Set a goal today of living and experiencing superior health, no matter how impossible it seems. Keep a child-like zest and zeal for life by chasing your dreams! By chasing your dreams, no matter how impossible they seem, you keep your mind and body youthful and you promote health. Even if your dream does not materialize, the fruit and reward is always the journey. By daily meditation you provide power and focus to your dreams. What you visualize you will realize!

Through the principles you learned in this book, the subjective experience of time slows down, and you will experience more present-moment awareness. This state creates more willpower, awareness, and more freedom to allow you to make the proper lifestyle choices and stick with them for the long-term. More importantly, this practice will engender long-term happiness and fulfillment. By practicing mindfulness, nutritional excellence, and exercise every day, you will experience joy and happiness in your everyday life. The end product, superior health, will manifest spontaneously. Embark on the journey to experience superior health and discover your true home, Satchitananda.

ENDNOTES

1. Gandhi, Mohandas K. (1993) *Gandhi: An Autobiography - The Story of My Experiments With Truth.* Boston: Beacon Press.

2. Brewer JA, Worhunsky PD, Gray JR, Tang Y-Y, Weber J, Kober H. Meditation experience is associated with differences in default mode network activity and connectivity. *Proceedings of the National Academy of Sciences of the United States of America.* 2011;108(50):20254-20259. doi:10.1073/pnas.1112029108.

About the Author

Dr. Orestes Gutierrez graduated from the Philadelphia College of Osteopathic Medicine. After serving in the Navy during the Iraq War, he completed Family Medicine training at the world-renowned Mayo Clinic. While a resident at Mayo Clinic Florida, he presented original research on exceptional longevity and nutrition internationally. The Florida Academy of Family Physicians awarded him its Distinguished Scholar Award in 2009. He currently has a private practice in Eugene, OR, holding dual board certification in Family Medicine and Integrative Holistic Medicine. As Assistant Clinical Professor of Family Medicine at Western and Pacific Northwest Universities, he is passionate about teaching clinical medicine and hosts medical student rotations. Most notably, Dr. Gutierrez practices the healthy lifestyle choices he recommends to his patients. He follows a whole-food, plant-based diet with his wife and children, practices Integral Yoga, and is an All-American Masters runner. He shares the knowledge he has gained through thirteen years of clinical practice and decades of personal practice in his first book.

Acknowledgements

I would like to thank all my mentors, teachers, and friends from FIU, PCOM, the US Navy, and Mayo Clinic Florida. There are too many to name and so many who have affected my path in life. Special recognition goes to Swami Jyotirmayananda from Yoga Research Foundation and Drs. Muata and Karen Ashby of the SEMA Institute for introducing me to authentic meditation and mindfulness practices. I am also grateful to the Unity communities of Jacksonville, FL and Eugene, OR for supporting my family's evolving spirituality. A special thanks to Lin and Robert of EVEN (Eugene Veg Education Network) for their continued endorsements. This book would not have been possible without supporting research completed by Maria Rose and Boone Gutierrez, and editing by Sofi and Pamela Gutierrez and Hadjer Bounama. And, finally, gratitude for my patients who have taught me so much and inspired me to write this book.

Made in the USA
San Bernardino, CA
21 November 2015